I0082742

FIBROMYALGIA UNRAVELED

YOUR GUIDE TO UNDERSTAND SYMPTOMS, NAVIGATE TREATMENT AND PRACTICE SELF-CARE

COURTNEY DALE

© **Copyright 2023 - All rights reserved.**

The content contained within this book may not be reproduced, duplicated or transmitted without direct written permission from the author or the publisher.

Under no circumstances will any blame or legal responsibility be held against the publisher, or author, for any damages, reparation, or monetary loss due to the information contained within this book, either directly or indirectly.

Legal Notice:

This book is copyright protected. It is only for personal use. You cannot amend, distribute, sell, use, quote or paraphrase any part, or the content within this book, without the consent of the author or publisher.

Disclaimer Notice:

Please note the information contained within this document is for educational and entertainment purposes only. All effort has been executed to present accurate, up to date, reliable, complete information. No warranties of any kind are declared or implied. Readers acknowledge that the author is not engaged in the rendering of legal, financial, medical or professional advice. The content within this book has been derived from various sources. Please consult a licensed professional before attempting any techniques outlined in this book.

By reading this document, the reader agrees that under no circumstances is the author responsible for any losses, direct or indirect, that are incurred as a result of the use of the information contained within this document, including, but not limited to, errors, omissions, or inaccuracies.

CONTENTS

INTRODUCTION

It's all in your head

Living life with fibromyalgia can be an incredibly challenging experience, to say the least. The frustration and pain that come with it are all too real, and it is essential to understand that fibromyalgia is most certainly not just "all in your head."

The phrase "It's all in your head" holds significant importance in recognizing its profound impact on mental health struggles. This statement has proven to be a formidable barrier for many, which stops them from seeking the help and insights and embracing true self-acceptance. The dismissive nature of this phrase can undermine the validity of your emotional and psychological experiences.

Many people living with fibromyalgia have had to face dismissive attitudes or misunderstandings from their friends, family, and even co-workers, who do not grasp the complexities of the seemingly "invisible illness." The time has come for you to acknowledge your struggles and feelings, as they are essential. You should never feel guilty about seeking empathy and support when you need it.

This book will discuss the misconception that fibromyalgia is merely psychological and stands firmly with you, offering you a compassionate and understanding perspective on your challenging journey.

It is important to acknowledge that the pain that you are constantly living with can result in mental health issues, which are real and can have tangible effects on one's health. Encouraging open conversations, empathy, and support can break down this barrier, fostering a more understanding and compassionate society where people are genuinely empowered to seek help and self-acceptance without judgment.

Introducing The LifeScape Technique, this book offers a range of strategies to cope with and manage the complexities of fibromyalgia. Throughout the subsequent chapters, these techniques will be discussed in depth, and you will be empowered to live a healthier life despite your struggle with fibromyalgia.

This book aims to provide you with facts, figures, and a genuine understanding of this condition's physical and emotional aspects. By delving into the scientific foundations and embracing empathy, the aim is to empower you, living with fibromyalgia, and your loved ones with the knowledge and compassion that is needed to navigate this challenging journey.

Light will be shed on the complexities of fibromyalgia, and you will be offered insights that foster empathy and support.

Yes, life can be challenging, and we all face unique problems, limitations, and pains. It is important to remember that you are never alone on your journey. Whether you are dealing with personal struggles, work-related stress, or other difficulties, seeking support and guidance is okay.

Remember, there is always hope for brighter days ahead when your world seems grey and gloomy. The reality is that you can overcome these obstacles by addressing your challenges head-on and actively seeking solutions that work for you. Don't ever hesitate to reach out to your friends, family, or professionals who can provide you with the support and understanding that you need.

It is important that you remind yourself every single day of your life just how resilient you are and that a brighter path is waiting for you.

The reason for buying a book like *Fibromyalgia Unraveled* varies from person to person. For many, it is a deep yearning for real answers and relief from the challenges of fibromyalgia.

It is that burning desperation and desire to understand your condition better and regain control of your life again. The hope of finally finding practical solutions and empathetic support. Whether you are on a quest for knowledge, comfort, or empowerment, this book serves as a beacon, shining light on the uncharted territory of fibromyalgia. It will speak to your unique journey, providing insight, guidance, and the companionship of understanding.

The lifescape technique is a transformative approach to personal growth. The following chapters will examine its strategies in detail. It is all about uncovering your full potential and enhancing well-being through mindfulness, goal setting, and self-discovery.

Fibromyalgia Unraveled is your path to a brighter, happier future where your symptoms are more manageable. Within the pages of this book, you will gain a profound understanding of your condition, a personalized roadmap to manage your symptoms, and a renewed sense of hope.

Imagine waking up each day with newfound energy, free from the shackles of constant agonizing pain. Picture a life where you are excited for each new day, where you are in control, can engage in activities you once loved, and relish restful nights.

This book aims to empower you to rebuild your life, strengthening not just your body but also your mind and spirit. By the final page, you will have the tools to embrace each day with a smile, knowing that a truly fulfilling life is within your reach.

The author's authority in this context is unquestionable and is an ideal guide for your journey. Their extensive expertise and unique insights have been developed through years of dedicated research and hands-on experience. The promised result was incredibly challenging, but the patience, work, and time were worth the author's groundbreaking revelations.

For many years, people have struggled due to the lack of access to new information which has the potential to revolutionize the way we approach fibromyalgia. With the guidance of the author, you can overcome previous difficulties and explore new territory with confidence and ease, leveraging their knowledge and expertise to achieve your goals.

If you have been seeking a book that resonates with empathy and understanding, *Fibromyalgia Unraveled* is the right choice. This insightful book goes beyond medical jargon to offer a warm, friendly hand in navigating the challenges of fibromyalgia. It provides a comforting companion for anyone desperately trying to manage this painful condition.

With its relatable stories, practical advice, and reassuring voice, it feels like a conversation with a close, trusted friend who truly gets what you are going through. *Fibromyalgia Unraveled* is more than a book; it is a source of support that will help you realize that you are not alone on your path.

Unraveling Fibromyalgia starts with a chapter that takes you through the vast array of symptoms associated with fibromyalgia and dispels common misconceptions. By the end of it, you will have a deep and clear understanding of fibromyalgia, helping you separate fact from fiction.

Next, you will dive into *The Language of the Body*. This chapter emphasizes the importance of tuning into your body and understanding its signals. Get ready to enhance your own ability to listen to your body's messages; it is like conversing with your own wellness.

Next up is *The Power of Pause*. This section highlights the significance of rest, relaxation, and quality sleep in managing fibromyalgia. You will find practical strategies to boost these aspects of your life, ensuring you experience rejuvenating rest and effective stress management.

Being hungry for knowledge makes the following chapter ideal. The chapter on the *Fibromyalgia-Food Connection* will help you explore the links between your diet and fibro symptoms. You will gain insights into how your dietary choices can impact your symptoms and discover actionable strategies for personalized nutrition.

In the chapter entitled *Movement and Medicine,* you will uncover the therapeutic potential of various movement modalities. This chapter aims to inspire you to find and embrace movement forms that align with your body's needs and preferences.

Now, let us create your sanctuary in *Your Sanctuary*. This section explores the profound influence of your environment on your well-being and symptom management. Learn practical strategies to design healing spaces and harness the therapeutic effects of nature.

Then we will move on to *Sounds That Heal,* which will be music to your ears! Here, you will dive into the transformative and therapeutic effects of music in managing fibromyalgia symptoms. You will also discover the science behind music therapy and create your personalized healing playlists.

Lastly, the chapter *Growth Amidst Pain* reminds you that living with any chronic condition can bring valuable life lessons. You will gain a brand new perspective on your condition and begin seeing fibromyalgia not just as a challenge but as a catalyst for personal growth and understanding.

Your journey through this book promises to be a friendlier and insightful experience. So, without further ado, let's get started by unraveling fibromyalgia.

1

UNRAVELING FIBROMYALGIA

L et's embark on an expedition into the very heart of fibromyalgia, breaking barriers and shining a light on the complexities that shape the experiences of those affected by this condition. In the maze of medical complexities, there exists a condition that often eludes clear comprehension: *fibromyalgia*.

This chronic pain condition is a puzzling enigma, challenging medical professionals and people battling its manifestations. To truly understand this condition is to embark on a journey through the multifaceted layers of pain, fatigue, and cognitive haze that define the daily existence of those affected.

Fibromyalgia isn't just a singular diagnosis; it is a tapestry of symptoms that interlace into a spectrum of experiences unique to each person. From the persistent ache that traverses the body to the cognitive cloudiness that blurs mental clarity, it is a condition that defies straightforward categorization.

In this chapter, we unravel the threads of fibromyalgia, revealing its core elements, the impact it casts upon daily life, and the myths clouding its perception. We will delve into the complex interplay of symptoms, causes, and challenges in diagnosis and treatment, painting a vivid picture of the realities faced by those living with this "invisible" illness.

Let's explore the reality of fibromyalgia, dispelling myths and stereotypes while providing insight from the medical perspective. Our goal is to educate and empower you with the knowledge and tools to navigate the complex landscape of fibromyalgia, improving your resilience and quality of life. Let's journey through this often misunderstood condition, shedding light on its truths and offering guidance for a brighter future.

WHAT IS FIBROMYALGIA?

Fibromyalgia is a condition that affects a significant number of people worldwide. It is a complex and chronic disorder that is characterized by amplified and widespread pain throughout various parts of your body. This pain is often accompanied by fatigue and cognitive difficulties, making day-to-day activities challenging.

Unlike temporary discomfort that goes away with time, fibromyalgia is persistent, pervasive, and long-lasting. The pain is not just a singular symptom but a confluence of sensations that affect muscles, tendons, and ligaments. This intricate interplay of symptoms can also make it challenging for professionals to diagnose and treat fibromyalgia effectively.

People with fibromyalgia often experience other symptoms in addition to pain, like difficulty sleeping, headaches, depression, and anxiety. These symptoms can further complicate the disorder and make it even more challenging to manage.

Despite the complexity of fibromyalgia, there are ways to manage the various symptoms and improve the quality of life for those with the condition. Treatment options include medication, lifestyle changes, and therapy, among others. While it may not always seem like it, with proper management, people with fibromyalgia can lead fulfilling and satisfying lives.

FIBROMYALGIA SYMPTOMS

Fibromyalgia is a condition that results in multiple regions of pain throughout the body. These regions often overlap with areas known as tender or trigger points, but not all of them are included. The pain associated with fibromyalgia is usually a consistent, dull ache that can be felt in four out of the five regions of pain as per the 2016 diagnostic criteria.

The current criteria refer to fibromyalgia pain as multisite pain, while in the past, it was defined as chronic, widespread pain. The diagnostic process now focuses on the location and severity of the pain, whereas in the past, the duration of pain was the main factor.

Primary Symptoms of Fibromyalgia

Living with fibromyalgia can significantly impact your quality of life due to pain, fatigue, and other persistent symptoms.

However, despite common misconceptions about the condition, there are ways to manage it effectively. Fibromyalgia causes a range of symptoms, including:

- **Widespread Pain:** The hallmark of fibromyalgia, this pervasive pain extends across the body, manifesting as aches, burning sensations, and throbbing discomfort in multiple areas.
- **Fatigue:** More than mere tiredness, this overwhelming fatigue impedes daily activities, leaving people drained and exhausted even after adequate rest.
- **Cognitive Challenges:** Better known as "fibro fog," this symptom entails difficulties with concentration, memory, and mental clarity, affecting the ability to focus and perform cognitive tasks effectively.

Secondary and Other Symptoms

Alongside the primary symptoms, people may experience a range of other manifestations like headaches, irritable bowel syndrome (IBS), restless legs syndrome, heightened sensitivity to touch, sound, or light, and disturbances in sleep patterns.

The presentation of symptoms in people with fibromyalgia can vary significantly. Some may experience heightened pain, while others might predominantly grapple with ongoing fatigue or cognitive challenges. This variability can often pose great challenges in the diagnosis and treatment of fibromyalgia.

FIBROMYALGIA DIAGNOSIS CHALLENGES

Diagnosing fibromyalgia is challenging due to its overlap with other conditions and the lack of a definitive test. Typically, a diagnosis of fibromyalgia currently involves an evaluation of symptoms, ruling out other conditions, and assessing specific tender points in the body.

Fibromyalgia is a condition that is often misunderstood and misdiagnosed. Here's an outline of the typical diagnosis process:

- **Medical History and Physical Examination:** Doctors start by discussing your medical history and symptoms and conducting a physical exam to check for tender points, muscle stiffness, and other signs associated with fibromyalgia.
- **Symptom Evaluation:** Fibromyalgia causes widespread pain and tenderness in specific areas so that doctors will ask about your symptoms. These symptoms help guide the diagnosis.
- **Exclusion of Other Conditions:** Since fibromyalgia symptoms mimic those of other conditions, such as rheumatoid arthritis, lupus, and chronic fatigue syndrome, doctors often perform tests to rule out these conditions. This may involve blood tests, imaging, and other diagnostic procedures.
- **Diagnostic Criteria:** Physicians use diagnostic criteria, such as the American College of Rheumatology's, which requires widespread pain lasting at least three months

and the presence of tender points. Doctors will make sure that you meet this diagnostic criteria before giving you a diagnosis of fibromyalgia.

- **Assessment of Widespread Pain:** A key feature of fibromyalgia is widespread pain across the body. Patients typically experience pain on both sides of the body, above and below the waist and along the spine.
- **Review of Other Symptoms:** Besides pain, doctors consider the presence of other symptoms like fatigue, sleep disturbances, headaches, irritable bowel syndrome, and cognitive issues, which are common in fibromyalgia.
- **Patient Input and Collaboration:** Patient involvement is crucial in the diagnosis. Sharing detailed information about symptoms and their impact on daily life helps in the diagnostic process.
- **Monitoring and Reevaluation:** As symptoms can vary over time, it's common for doctors to want to monitor and reevaluate the condition periodically. This helps in adjusting treatment plans and ensuring the most effective management.
- **Multidisciplinary Approach:** A combination of healthcare professionals like rheumatologists, neurologists, and pain specialists might be involved in the diagnosis and treatment to address the diverse symptoms of fibromyalgia.

Remember, the process of diagnosing fibromyalgia is often based on the elimination of other conditions and the recognition of a specific set of symptoms. It is a collaborative effort between the patient and the healthcare team, focusing on managing symptoms and improving the patient's quality of life.

CAUSES AND RISK FACTORS OF FIBROMYALGIA

Many people often need clarification on the terms "causes" and "risk factors." Causes are the actual cause of a condition. Whereas risk factors are certain factors that may increase your likelihood of developing fibromyalgia.

Firstly, let us start off by having a look at the common causes of fibromyalgia. Thus far, it has been determined that some of the causes of fibromyalgia include:

Physical or Emotional Events: Physical trauma or emotional stress can sometimes act as triggering events for the onset of fibromyalgia symptoms. Trauma, such as injuries from accidents or surgeries, and ongoing emotional stressors are believed to exacerbate or initiate fibromyalgia symptoms potentially.

Infection: Infection to exacerbate or initiate fibromyalgia symptoms potentially. Some studies propose that infections or illnesses, particularly those affecting the immune system, might act as triggers for fibromyalgia in some people. These can include viral infections or other microbial agents.

Next, we are going to have a look at what increases a person's likelihood of developing fibromyalgia. Some common risk factors when it comes to fibromyalgia include:

- **Sex:** Fibromyalgia is more prevalent in women than in men. The reasons for this gender disparity are not entirely understood, but hormonal, genetic, and societal factors might contribute.
- **Family History:** A significant risk factor is having a family history of fibromyalgia. If a close relative, such as a parent or sibling, has the condition, there might be an increased likelihood of developing it.
- **Genetics:** Genetic predisposition appears to also play a role in the development of fibromyalgia. Research indicates that specific genetic mutations or variations may increase susceptibility to this condition. However, it is not solely determined by genetics and likely involves a complex interplay of genetic and environmental factors.
- **Other Disorders:** People living with certain other health conditions, such as rheumatic diseases, lupus, or osteoarthritis, seem to have a higher risk of developing fibromyalgia. People with depression or anxiety also have higher rates of fibromyalgia.

Understanding these potential causes and risk factors helps in both the diagnosis and management of fibromyalgia. However, as research progresses, the complexities and interactions among these factors continue to be studied, offering hope for improved treatments and more personalized approaches to managing this condition.

MEDICAL TREATMENT AND BEYOND

How To Treat Fibromyalgia

At the moment, there is no known cure for fibromyalgia. When you first get diagnosed and find out that there is no cure, this can be a scary moment. However, the focus of treatment revolves around easing symptoms and enhancing quality of life through a range of approaches, including medications, self-care strategies, and lifestyle adjustments.

Managing fibromyalgia involves a comprehensive approach. Medications like pain relievers, antiseizure drugs, and antidepressants are usually prescribed to help alleviate fibromyalgia symptoms. Additionally, various therapeutic interventions like physical therapy and cognitive-behavioral therapy form crucial components of managing the condition.

For pain relief and improved sleep, medications that are commonly prescribed include:

- pain relievers
- antiseizure drugs
- antidepressants

Pain relievers that are often prescribed include:

- acetaminophen
- aspirin
- ibuprofen

- naproxen

These medications can help you by reducing any discomfort and improving your ability to manage daily activities. It is important to consult a healthcare professional to discuss pain management options.

While nonsteroidal anti-inflammatory drugs (NSAIDs) may be useful for pain relief, they carry potential side effects, particularly with prolonged use. Caution is necessary when considering these drugs for chronic pain management.

Opioids have been used for pain relief, but studies have not shown consistent long-term effectiveness and can pose health risks due to increasing dosages over time.

Antiseizure drugs like pregabalin and gabapentin, as well as certain antidepressants such as duloxetine and milnacipran, have shown promise in managing pain and fatigue associated with fibromyalgia.

Furthermore, there are ongoing investigations into experimental treatments for fibromyalgia. There are natural remedies that aim to reduce stress and alleviate pain in conjunction with medical treatments like:

- acupuncture
- massage therapy
- meditation
- journaling
- exercise

- different therapies, including cognitive behavioral therapy (CBT)
- group therapy

It is important to note that managing your stress is vitally important, as stress can trigger fibromyalgia symptom flare-ups. If you are considering alternative therapies, be open and honest with your healthcare provider. It is always best to talk to your healthcare provider about them, as many remedies have not been extensively studied or proven effective.

THE IMPACT OF FIBROMYALGIA

Fibromyalgia is an incredibly complex disorder that affects your physical, mental, and emotional health. In fact, determining cause and effect when it comes to this complex illness can be tricky, but understanding these links has helped us better treat the problem from many different angles.

Since fibromyalgia is such a complex and multifaceted disorder, it can be challenging to determine the exact cause and effect of its symptoms. However, understanding the various relationships between the different factors that contribute to the development of fibromyalgia can help to develop more effective treatments. By addressing the physical, emotional, and psychological aspects of the disorder, healthcare professionals can offer more comprehensive care to patients.

Moreover, research has shown that lifestyle changes, such as regular exercise, stress management techniques, and sleep hygiene, can be effective in reducing the symptoms of fibromyalgia (Phillips, 2022). As such, a holistic approach that addresses the different aspects of the disorder can be beneficial in managing fibromyalgia and improving the quality of life for those who suffer from it.

How Does Fibromyalgia Affect Your Mental Health

Fibromyalgia can significantly affect your emotional well-being, although it is trickier to measure its full impact. Living with constant pain, battling fatigue, and struggling to concentrate can leave you feeling emotionally exhausted. Many people facing fibromyalgia find themselves isolated due to the challenges they experience in daily functioning and finding joy.

The constant effort to maintain a cheerful outlook can be overwhelming. While this doesn't always lead to diagnosed mental health disorders like depression or anxiety, the emotional toll is considerable.

To add to the complexity, fibromyalgia can exacerbate in response to stress or emotional burdens, creating a blurred connection between the condition and your emotional health. It's a two-way street where one can influence the other, making it challenging to distinguish between the two.

The Profound Impact of Fibromyalgia

Claire's Story

Claire's journey with fibromyalgia is a labyrinth of challenges, a poignant tale woven from real-life experiences mirrored in the lives of many people grappling with this condition. Fibromyalgia touched every aspect of Claire's life: physically, socially, emotionally, and psychologically.

Physical Challenges

Each morning, Claire awakens, greeted not by the promise of a new day but by the familiarity of relentless pain. It is a symphony of discomfort that courses through her body, ranging from a dull, persistent ache to sharp, piercing sensations. Every step is a testament to her resilience, as her muscles protest even the simplest movements, and the weight of fatigue presses upon her shoulders like an unwelcome burden. With each step that she takes, it feels as though her ankles want to break. However, despite the physical pain, Claire pushes herself forward with every bit of inner strength she has.

Social and Emotional Toll

The isolation woven by the threads of her symptoms becomes evident as the day progresses. Claire, once a vivacious socialite, now navigates the world with caution, for the vibrancy of her social life has dimmed. The invitations she once joyously accepted are now met with hesitation.

Clare manages her energy reserves to meet daily demands. As she distances herself from events, the tendrils of isolation subtly tighten.

The emotional landscape mirrors the unpredictability of her symptoms.

There are days when she attempts to seize control, yet the ebbs and flows of pain and fatigue, seemingly beyond her command, render her plans futile. The pervasive frustration and sadness cast shadows across her spirit, obscuring the brightness that once defined her essence.

Psychological Nuances

The invisible battle within Clare's mind is as arduous as the physical struggles. The fibrofog that envelops her thoughts often muddles up even the simplest tasks, leaving her grasping for words or losing the conversation thread. The once-sharp mind now navigates a maze of confusion and memory lapses, fostering a sense of inadequacy and self-doubt.

Yet, amidst the shadows, there are glimmers of resilience. Claire, armed with the unwavering support of her loved ones, finds solace in small victories – the gentle touch of under-standing from her partner, the unwavering companionship of her loyal pet, and the warmth of the community she has discov-ered within online support groups.

Insights Into the Fibromyalgia Experience

Claire's story stands as the perfect example of the diverse set of challenges that people with fibromyalgia face daily. Fibromyalgia is an affliction that causes chronic symptoms that can be debilitating and make even the most basic of tasks seem impossible.

In Claire's case, her story reflects not only the physical impedi-ments but also the emotional and psychological intricacies that come with the condition. Despite the constant pain and the overwhelming sense of fatigue, Claire perseveres. Her story is a source of inspiration for many others who have fibromyalgia, as it shows that even in the darkest of times, there is always hope. It is a story of resilience, strength, and courage.

The condition is often invisible, with no visible symptoms which can make it difficult for others to understand the extent of the pain and suffering felt by those who have it. However, Claire's story sheds light on the often-unseen struggles of people with fibromyalgia, and her example reminds us that despite the challenges, there is always hope to overcome them.

DEBUNKING COMMON MISCONCEPTIONS ABOUT FIBROMYALGIA

Fibromyalgia is subject to numerous misconceptions that can lead to confusion and skepticism. Addressing these misunderstandings is crucial in supporting those grappling with this complex condition.

Debunking these misconceptions is vital in fostering understanding, empathy, and better support for people navigating the challenges of fibromyalgia. Recognizing the realities of this condition enables a more compassionate and informed approach to its management and treatment.

Let us have a look at a few of the common misconceptions about fibromyalgia.

Myth 1: It Isn't a Real Disorder

The Truth: Fibromyalgia is indeed a real and recognized medical condition. Though its diagnosis may be challenging due to the complexity of its symptoms, the pain, fatigue, and cognitive difficulties experienced by those living with this invisible illness are very real.

Myth 2: Fibromyalgia Is a 'Catchall' Diagnosis

The Truth: Fibromyalgia is a distinct condition characterized by specific symptoms such as widespread pain, fatigue, and cognitive challenges. It is not merely a general diagnosis when other conditions cannot be identified. Its diagnosis is based on a combination of different symptoms and a clinical assessment.

Myth 3: Fibromyalgia Only Affects Women

The Truth: While fibromyalgia is more common among women, it can affect any gender. Men can also experience this condition, albeit less frequently, potentially leading to under-diagnosis or delayed diagnosis due to the misconception that it exclusively affects women.

Myth 4: There's Nothing You Can Do

The Truth: People can manage fibromyalgia despite the absence of a cure. Lifestyle adjustments, therapies, and various strategies can significantly improve symptoms and quality of life.

Myth 5: Complementary and Alternative Treatments Are Pointless

The Truth: While not curative, complementary treatments like acupuncture, massage therapy, and certain dietary modifications may help in managing symptoms and improving overall well-being for some people with fibromyalgia.

Myth 6: You Should Avoid Exercise

The Truth: Exercise is a vital part of managing fibromyalgia. While it's important to find the right balance and type of exercise that suits your needs, gentle physical activity can improve strength, flexibility, and overall well-being.

Myth 7: You're Just Tired

The Truth: Fatigue in fibromyalgia is not simply feeling tired; it's an overwhelming, persistent feeling of exhaustion that significantly impacts daily activities and is not alleviated by rest.

Myth 8: You Can Take a Pill to Make Fibromyalgia Symptoms Disappear

The Truth: No pill magically eradicates fibromyalgia. Medications can help manage symptoms, but a comprehensive approach involving various strategies is necessary to improve quality of life.

Myth 9: You Must Have Tender Points to Have Fibromyalgia

The Truth: Tender points were previously used as part of the diagnostic criteria, but the current diagnostic guidelines do not necessitate the presence of tender points to diagnose fibromyalgia. Diagnosis is now primarily symptom-based.

Myth 10: Fibromyalgia and Arthritis are the Same Conditions

The Truth: Fibromyalgia is often confused with arthritis due to the shared symptom of pain. However, they are very distinct conditions. Arthritis primarily involves joint inflammation, while fibromyalgia is more about widespread pain, muscle tenderness, and other symptoms like fatigue and cognitive challenges.

By dispelling these myths, a more accurate understanding of fibromyalgia can be fostered. It is a complex condition that warrants a multifaceted approach to management and support for those navigating its challenges.

Understanding the reality of fibromyalgia is crucial in providing empathy, support, and appropriate care for people affected by this condition.

In this chapter, *Unraveling Fibro*, we embarked on an exploration of the complexities surrounding fibromyalgia. We defined this chronic condition, highlighting its widespread pain, fatigue, and cognitive challenges.

Additionally, we explored the variability in symptom presentation among people, discussing the potential causes, risk factors, diagnostic challenges, and the medical approach to managing this condition. Addressing prevalent myths, we debunked misconceptions, emphasizing the multifaceted nature of fibromyalgia and its significant impact on the lives of those affected.

Continuing our journey, we delve into a profound connection: *The Language of the Body,* beyond the overt symptoms and diagnoses, our bodies communicate in intricate ways, revealing underlying stories often unheard or misunderstood. In the context of fibromyalgia, understanding this silent dialogue between the body and the self can offer unique insights and strategies.

The upcoming chapter aims to unravel these subtleties, exploring how listening to the body's language can provide a deeper understanding of managing and coping with chronic conditions like fibromyalgia. From physical manifestations to emotional responses, we will decipher this unspoken language, empowering people to form a more profound relationship with their bodies and enhance their well-being.

2

THE LANGUAGE OF THE BODY

There's a Cherokee proverb, "Pay attention to the whispers, so we won't have to listen to the screams."

Your body is ready to communicate with you, and it's time to become aware of what it's saying. The reality is that your body constantly communicates with you, sending subtle signals with great wisdom that can change your life. The question is, are you attuned enough to hear your body's whispers before they become cries and screams?

Every day, your body orchestrates an incredible orchestra of sensations, feelings, and whispers. It is like a silent conversation that carries insights into your well-being.

In this chapter, you will embark on a journey to discover why lending an attentive ear to your body's messages is so important. When you have fibromyalgia, you must be in tune with the language of your body. When you can interpret the cues and signals it sends you, you are well on your way to managing your fibromyalgia.

By the end of this chapter, you will know precisely why listening to your body and learning from it can be a life-changing practice. So, sit back and get ready to dive into the marvelous world of fibromyalgia body awareness.

Health Challenges? Not Listening To Your Body Is Costing You

Every now and then, life and your body communicate with you subtly, like a whisper in the wind. Other times, it's as direct as a bold billboard right before us! The key is to tune in to those subtle signals and prevent those sudden, in-your-face moments.

It is always important to listen to your body, especially if you are facing health challenges. Ignoring your body's signals can cost you time, money, and happiness. Pushing through and pretending everything's fine just because you want to be strong might not be the best approach, especially when you have fibromyalgia.

Remember that real strength and power come from acknowledging that a health challenge affects your life. It is not about being an unsung hero but about accepting where you are right now. This acceptance is your vantage point for making positive changes that support your well-being and your in a healthier way.

Listening to your body is a bit like gathering puzzle pieces, taking in the data it provides, and then making wise choices for your well-being. When juggling the responsibilities of getting through your daily commitments and managing a health challenge, being in sync with your body's messages becomes crucial.

It is super important that you pay attention to these signals, as ignoring them can result in serious and unfavorable outcomes. Don't let the consequences catch you off guard - stay alert and heed any warning signs your body is sending you.

Listening to your body's signals will pave the way for a harmonious connection between your mind and physical well-being. This will empower you to confidently make more informed decisions, foster a deeper understanding of your needs, and ultimately lead you toward a path of holistic health and greater vitality.

Tuning into and listening to your body will:

- Empower your inner compass and self-awareness & boost your confidence. When you trust your inner wisdom and follow your intuition, you nurture a deep sense of self-assurance. This self-assurance will give you the unwavering belief that you truly understand yourself.
- Discover Inner Serenity. Having faith in your ability to listen to your body's signals brings you an inner peace that assures you'll recognize your limits and when to take a step back before any issues arise.
- Say Goodbye to Flare-Ups, Fatigue, and Discomfort. By listening closely to your body's messages, you can identify what actions to take or avoid early on, making informed choices for your well-being. By reducing the

occurrence of flare-ups, fatigue, pain, or other symptoms, you'll find yourself more efficient and dependable on yourself.

8 TYPES OF FIBROMYALGIA PAIN

Living life with such a painful chronic condition like fibromyalgia can be stressful, and it is not surprising that fibromyalgia warriors are emotionally and mentally exhausted. Currently, about 2% of adults in the US live with fibromyalgia (FMS), according to the Centers for Disease Control and Prevention.

Due to the nature of the disease and the challenges that accompany FMS, it is also associated with an increased risk of suicide. Various studies have shown that between 27% and 58% of people with fibromyalgia understandably report feeling depressed, hopeless, and even thoughts of suicide.

Researchers believe that the nervous systems of people who are living with fibromyalgia are overly sensitive to pain.

There are eight main types of fibromyalgia (FMS) pain. If you have fibromyalgia, you'll likely experience several of them if you have this condition.

The different types of fibromyalgia pain include:

- Allodynia
- Digestive pain
- Headaches
- Hyperalgesia

- Neuropathic pain
- Pelvic pain
- Temporomandibular joint pain (TMJ)
- Widespread muscle pain and fatigue

Let us look at these different types of pain and how they can be treated.

Allodynia

Allodynia is skin pain caused by central sensitization. This type of pain can make even a light touch hurt. Nociceptors, the nerves that detect sensations, can become over-sensitive, causing normal sensations to be interpreted as pain. Lyrica (pregabalin) can help treat allodynia in people with FMS.

Digestive Pain

Fibromyalgia affects up to 70% of people with IBS, causing headaches and migraines. Treatment options include medication and avoiding triggers. IBS causes cramping, pain, constipation, diarrhea, and nausea. Acid reflux is also common in people with fibromyalgia. Fibromyalgia sufferers are more likely to have chronic GERD, a chronic form of acid reflux. Treatment includes lifestyle changes, medication, and dietary adjustments.

Headaches

Tension headaches cause a dull, tightening sensation all around the head, while migraines are more painful and typically occur on one side of the head with light and sound sensitivity. A 2018 study found that migraines are more severe in people with fibromyalgia. Treatment includes prescription medications like triptans and NSAIDs and avoiding triggers.

Hyperalgesia

Hyperalgesia is a condition where fibromyalgia patients feel increased pain sensitivity. Researchers found that women with fibromyalgia had tissues around their muscles that were hyper-reactive to even light touches. In contrast, muscle activity was similar in healthy women and women with chronic fatigue syndrome. The researchers believe that the nervous systems of women with fibromyalgia send signals that keep the tissues in a heightened state of alert.

Neuropathic Pain

Neuropathic pain causes crawling, tingling, or burning sensations in the arms and legs. Prescription treatments and over-the-counter creams like capsaicin or lidocaine can help ease the pain. Some studies suggest that vitamin B1, B6, and B12 supplements may help with neuropathic pain.

Pelvic Pain

Women with endometriosis may experience pelvic and abdominal pain, frequent urination, and bladder pain if they also have fibromyalgia. A 2019 study shows that women with endometriosis also have a 6% higher chance of developing fibromyalgia.

- Endometriosis treatment options include:
- hormonal therapies
- complementary treatments

- lifestyle changes
- surgical procedures, including a hysterectomy

Temporomandibular Joint Pain

FMS often causes TMJ pain, a dull ache felt in the jaw, ear, temple, eyes, lower jaw, or neck. Dentists diagnose TMJ and might suggest wearing a mouth guard to prevent teeth grinding. Anti-inflammatory drugs like Aleve or Advil can help, and muscle relaxants or FMS pain drugs can be prescribed if the pain persists.

Widespread Muscle Pain

Widespread muscle pain is the hallmark of fibromyalgia and can make you feel like you have the flu or even hurt all over. A lot of people with fibromyalgia also tend to have:

- Pain between your shoulder blades
- Lower back pain, which can spread into the buttocks and legs
- Breastbone and rib cage pain that feels like a heart attack
- Neck and back pain that moves into the shoulders

Three drugs commonly used to ease the pain and discomfort of fibromyalgia pain include:

- Cymbalta
- Savella
- Lyrica

It is also important to know that physical therapy and exercises, like yoga, walking, or swimming, can also help reduce pain levels and loosen the muscles and joints. Other lifestyle choices like reducing your stress levels and prioritizing sleep can also help manage pain.

There are no two ways about it. Living with fibromyalgia is not for the faint-hearted, and it is hard to live with it, especially when the symptoms and painful attacks can be so unpredictable.

It is, however, not all doom and gloom because by investing time and patience into experimenting with different treatments, it is possible to find relief from the symptoms of FMS. Additionally, several mobile health-tracking apps can help you monitor and document your symptoms, diet, activity, pain levels, and more.

Some mobile apps that you can try include:

MyFitnessPal: Helps you to track your daily calorie intake, exercise, and weight management goals.

Samsung Health: Monitors your daily activities, exercise, and sleep and provides personalized insights and wellness programs.

Apple Health: A comprehensive health app for iOS devices that tracks various health metrics, including activity, sleep, nutrition, and more.

Google Fit: Tracks your daily activity, heart rate, and step count and integrates with other fitness apps and devices.

Lifesum: Helps you track your food intake, set nutrition and weight loss goals, and provides personalized meal plans.

MyNetDiary: Tracks your food intake exercise and offers features like barcode scanning, meal planning, and nutrient intake analysis.

Health Mate: A health and fitness tracking app that monitors your activity, sleep, and weight and enables easy health metrics tracking.

Please note that availability and features may vary depending on the platform (iOS, Android) that you are using and the country that you are in. It's always a good idea to read reviews and check the app's features before choosing one that suits your unique needs.

Feel free to research, as there are many different tools available out there that can help you. Remember that all of these factors influence your pain levels and overall well-being.

THE CONCEPT OF FEEDBACK

In the context of the body, feedback loops play an important role in maintaining balance and regulating various physiological processes. Feedback loops involve continuously monitoring and adjusting certain variables within your body to maintain homeostasis, which is the body's stable internal environment.

In the case of fibromyalgia and other chronic conditions, understanding the body's feedback loops can be beneficial for recognizing triggers, understanding symptom flare-ups, and devising strategies to restore balance. Let us take stress and fibromyalgia as an example.

Stress can greatly contribute to fibromyalgia symptoms, setting off a feedback loop where pain increases stress, leading to further increases in pain. This feedback loop can create a cycle where the symptoms worsen over time. Recognizing and intervening in these loops becomes essential for managing the condition effectively.

People can implement strategies to interrupt this feedback loop and restore balance by recognizing the relationship between stress and fibromyalgia symptoms. This might involve stress management techniques like:

- relaxation exercises
- stress reduction activities
- seeking support from healthcare professionals.

By breaking the cycle of stress amplifying symptoms and symptoms amplifying stress, people have a better chance of managing and minimizing the impact of fibromyalgia. Understanding the feedback loops within the body allows people to identify the connections between different variables, such as stress and symptoms, and develop personalized strategies to intervene in these loops. Through targeted interventions, you can strive to restore balance, reduce symptom severity, and improve your overall well-being.

The main point of this chapter is the importance of effective communication through body language. It explored how your non-verbal cues can greatly impact the message you convey. By knowing your body language and understanding its impact, you can enhance your communication skills and better connect with others.

Remember that when you have fibromyalgia, your body speaks and screams at you in its own unique way. When you have overexerted yourself too much, been neglecting your sleep routine or diet, and when you have been stressed out.

ARE YOU LISTENING TO YOUR BODY?

Did you know that your body always tries to communicate with you and is like a friendly companion? If you listen closely, your body will guide you in various aspects of your life, including in managing fibromyalgia.

Listening to your body will help you know when you need to rest, push yourself harder, or be still and recharge. The only challenge is that many of us still need to learn the art of listening to our bodies.

From a young age, we tend to overlook its signals, numbing uncomfortable sensations with painkillers. We push ourselves, ignore exhaustion, and dismiss the whispers and warnings it sends us through various means, like illness or discomfort. Sometimes, we miss those subtle cues, and our bodies respond with stronger signals that demand immediate attention.

Your body is amazing and intuitive, and it will nudge you towards spending time with the right people and avoiding those who may not be a positive influence. Your body also knows what work aligns best with your inner self and where to direct your efforts. It is like a futuristic GPS for life that is constantly connected, suggesting the right paths and routes.

In reality, your body holds a profound intelligence, going much deeper than the mind can comprehend. It speaks to you in a multitude of ways. So, are you listening? Do you know how to tune in to this friendly source of wisdom and guidance?

It is fascinating to think about how your body constantly communicates with you. From the obvious signals like pain or hunger to the more subtle cues like fatigue, mood swings, and specific cravings, it is as if your body lets you know what it needs and how you are doing. It is like a continuous conversation between you and your incredible biological machine.

Mindful Listening in a Noisy World

Have you ever noticed how your thoughts can get jumbled when you are surrounded by noise and distractions? This question really hits home, especially in today's modern world. Noise and distractions can come from all angles - blaring car horns, sirens, or even the chaos in the hallway just outside your office door.

Sometimes, it is not the external noise but your own inner monologue, constantly chattering away, giving you a hard time. And in this modern age, with all the time spent on social media and inundated with the news, it often feels like there is more yelling and arguing than any genuine listening or understanding.

But here's the thing: you are not just hearing an annoying sound when you hear noise. You are hearing something loaded with meaning. It could be a feeling of annoyance, resistance, or even a sense of threat. All this noise makes it tough to focus because it is like a signal that your thoughts are under siege, and you feel like you are being attacked. And interestingly, it is not always an external foe - often, it is your internal thoughts and feelings clamoring for attention.

This is not just limited to the workplace or school, though. It also happens in your personal life, especially when you are trying to meditate, practice mindfulness, or concentrate on a task. One noise, even a tiny one, can shatter your concentration and drain your energy levels. So, what is the solution?

When the World Is Too Noisy, What Can You Do?

When the world gets a bit too noisy, instead of letting frustration take over and shouting at the racket, try this: Take a deep breath and listen. Embrace the act of listening with curiosity and an open heart - maybe even a touch of compassion.

Pay closer attention to your reactions rather than fixating on the sounds themselves. Observe your response without any self-judgment or internal commentary. By doing this, you will be fully present in the moment and find that your mind begins to quiet down.

It is true that some sounds naturally trigger a heightened response due to our biologies, like a loud bang or someone screaming. These can startle you, making your heart race and causing you to flinch. However, it is important to recognize that noise is not just about the quality of the sound itself; it is equally about how we respond to it.

Practicing Awareness of The Sound and Silence

Sound is all around us, but how aware are you of the different sounds that are around you? You can use this simple exercise to start attuning yourself more to the sounds of the world around you.

Find a comfortable sitting position, close your eyes, and begin to focus on your own awareness. Take a moment to observe the nature of your awareness. Is it clear or a bit fuzzy? Does it remain steady or come and go?

If you hear any sounds around you, pay close attention to them. See if you can discern any rhythm in the sounds and how your body responds to them. Do you feel tension or relaxation as these sounds emerge and subside? Notice where tension may reside in your body - perhaps in your forehead, mouth, shoulders, or stomach.

And don't forget the importance of your thoughts. Thoughts are just the mind doing its thing, and that's perfectly fine. Sensations, however, are your body's way of being. If your mind starts to wander, it's alright. You are aware of it, and that's what matters. Gently guide your focus back to your awareness.

Have you ever noticed a moment when there's a sound, but it's not disruptive? Or a precious moment of silence between the sounds? Take a deep breath and appreciate how the sound actually highlights the beauty of the silence, and the silence enhances the richness of the sounds.

As you practice this, you'll find that your mind transitions from battling the sounds to being open and receptive. Instead of feeling restless or irritated, you may even discover a sense of calm and joy in the process.

Mindful Listening Throughout The Day

You can incorporate mindful listening into your daily routine, especially when something disrupts or diverts your focus from what you'd rather be doing. Instead of letting pain, worries, or frustration consume you, try this:

1. Close your eyes for a moment, take two deep breaths, and pay attention to what's around you or any sounds in the environment.
2. As you inhale, be mindful of your reactions to your surroundings. Take note of any passing thoughts or thought patterns in your mind. Observe whether your breathing is becoming faster or slower and if there are moments of silence between breaths.
3. Take a deep breath, and gently shift your focus to boost your thinking skills. Pay attention to how you feel afterward.

You can apply this practice at home when conversing with your loved ones, whether they're your children, spouse, or parents.

It's also helpful in an office setting, whether you're dealing with co-workers or your boss.

When you tune into your moment-to-moment reactions to whatever comes your way, you better understand how your mind operates. This practice boosts your thinking skills, making deciphering the significance of what you encounter easier. What used to be noise that grated on your nerves transforms into a sound you can listen to and assess. Rather than harboring frustration towards the world, you feel more at ease within it.

As you openly explore the workings of your mind, you will find that openness becomes a defining trait of your thought process, allowing the world to unveil its true depth and clarity.

By learning to listen to, interpret, and use your body's signals, you can learn to understand your body's needs and cater to them more effectively. The next chapter is entitled *The Power of Pause*. Hold onto your seat because this adventure is going to be an exciting and informative one.

3

THE POWER OF PAUSE

> Activity and rest are two vital aspects of life. To find a balance in them is a skill in itself. Wisdom is knowing when to have rest, when to have activity, and how much of each to have.

— SRI SRI RAVI SHANKAR

Just like many others, young Clarise was struggling to manage her fibromyalgia symptoms. Her days were filled with constant fatigue and aches that seemed to seep into every fiber of her being.

Clarise would wake up every day exhausted, feeling like she had run a marathon while sleeping. Despite her overwhelming tiredness, she summoned every ounce of strength to get out of bed and face the day's challenges.

Before Clarise was diagnosed with fibromyalgia, she realized that even the simplest daily tasks were monumental challenges. Every step felt like walking through quicksand, and her body weighed her down with an invisible force. Each movement sent waves of pain through her muscles, leaving her feeling helpless and frustrated.

Clarise had always been an active person, full of life and energy. But, her world had been reduced to a constant battle against the overwhelming fatigue that fibromyalgia brought. It felt like she was trapped in a body that no longer belonged to her, a body that betrayed her at every turn.

The fatigue often hit her in waves, leaving Clarise unable to predict when or how it would strike. Some days, it would come crashing down upon her like a tidal wave, rendering her bedridden and unable to function. On other days, it would linger in the background, a constant reminder of her limitations.

Despite the challenges, Clarise refused to give up. She sought support from fellow fibromyalgia patients and connected with online communities where she found solace in knowing she wasn't alone. She learned to embrace the power of pausing, pacing herself, listening to her body's signals, and adjusting her activities accordingly.

Through it all, Clarise's spirit remained resilient. She may have been fighting an invisible battle, but she refused to let fibromyalgia define her. With each passing day, she learned to adapt, embrace the moments of rest, and appreciate the small victories. She became an advocate, raising awareness about fibromyalgia and the debilitating fatigue that comes with it.

Clarise's story serves as a reminder of fibromyalgia warriors' strength and determination. Despite indescribably painful challenges, fibromyalgia warriors continue to push forward, fighting for better days and a brighter future.

When you have fibromyalgia, it is essential to get the rest that your body needs to avoid those nasty flare-ups where your body is screaming at you. So many fibromyalgia warriors are not in attunement to the signals that their body is sending, or they want to push through the pain and get the things done that they need to do. Either way, the power of pause can help fibro warriors improve their quality of life.

Have you ever taken the time to reflect on the power of pausing? The power of pause is about being gentle with yourself and giving your body the time it needs to rest and recuperate. It's important to remember that rest is not just about physical rest but also mental and emotional rejuvenation. Integrating pauses into your daily routine can make a significant difference in managing the everyday challenges of fibromyalgia.

This chapter will help you to embrace the power that exists in the power of pause so that you can use it to improve your overall well-being.

THE RELATIONSHIP BETWEEN FIBROMYALGIA AND FATIGUE

Musculoskeletal pain, tenderness, and fatigue are all symptoms of fibromyalgia. Abnormal pain signal processing in the nervous system disrupts sleep and energy metabolism, leading to persistent exhaustion. Other symptoms, such as muscle stiffness, cognitive difficulties, and mood disturbances, contribute to fatigue.

Managing fatigue requires symptom management, lifestyle adjustments, and self-care, such as regular exercise and stress reduction techniques. It is important to recognize the debilitating impact of fatigue on daily functioning and overall well-being.

The relationship between fibromyalgia and fatigue is complex and multifaceted, and the two often go hand in hand. Here are some key points that are important for you to understand:

1. **Fatigue as a primary symptom:** Fatigue is one of the primary symptoms of fibromyalgia. The feeling is often described as persistent and overwhelming tiredness that does not improve with rest or sleep. This fatigue can significantly impact daily functioning, productivity, and quality of life.

2. **Chronic fatigue syndrome (CFS):** Fibromyalgia shares similarities with chronic fatigue syndrome (CFS), and the two conditions often overlap. Many people with fibromyalgia also experience symptoms of long-lasting fatigue characteristic of CFS.

3. **Sleep disturbances:** Sleep disturbances are common in fibromyalgia and can contribute to the experience of fatigue. People living with fibromyalgia often struggle with falling asleep, staying asleep, or experiencing restful sleep. The disrupted sleep patterns can worsen fatigue levels and perpetuate a cycle of sleep deprivation and exhaustion.

4. **Pain-fatigue cycle:** Fibromyalgia is associated with widespread pain. The pain experienced can lead to physical and emotional fatigue. Conversely, fatigue can make pain feel more intense, creating a vicious cycle known as the pain-fatigue cycle.

5. **Reduced exercise tolerance:** Fatigue can make exercising or performing physical activity difficult. Reduced exercise tolerance can lead to deconditioning and further exacerbate fatigue levels.

6. **Central nervous system dysfunction:** Research suggests that fibromyalgia may involve dysfunction in the central nervous system, leading to amplified sensations, including fatigue. This dysfunction can also affect sleep regulation, pain perception, and energy levels.

7. **Mental and emotional factors:** Fibromyalgia is commonly associated with mental and emotional factors such as depression, anxiety, and stress. These factors can contribute to fatigue and make it more challenging to manage.

Living with fibromyalgia means that you need to address fatigue and develop coping strategies that really work for you. This may include:

- pacing your daily activities
- managing your stress levels
- practicing good sleep hygiene
- adopting daily relaxation techniques
- engaging in gentle exercise
- seeking support from healthcare professionals

Understanding the relationship between fibromyalgia and fatigue can help you navigate your symptoms and find effective strategies to manage your energy levels and improve overall well-being.

ENERGY-OPTIMIZING ROUTINES FOR FIBROMYALGIA WARRIORS

When you have a chronic health condition like fibromyalgia, it is important that you carefully manage your energy reserves so that you can maintain your physical and mental well-being. Energy currency is a term that is used to describe the limited amount of energy available to people with chronic conditions. Due to your health condition, you must be cautious about how much energy you expend during the day, as overexertion can lead to exhaustion and worsening of your symptoms.

To manage your energy currency, you must plan your day carefully and always consider your energy requirements and personal goals. You must pace yourself and prioritize your activities based on your energy levels. This means that you will need to allocate your energy resources efficiently, focusing on the most important tasks and avoiding activities that require a lot of energy.

Optimizing your daily functioning will help you avoid overexertion, which can worsen your symptoms. By understanding and applying the concept of energy currency in your life, you can better control your chronic condition and improve your overall quality of life. This will help you to strike a good balance between managing your symptoms and achieving your goals.

Never forget that no matter your pain levels, there is always hope for a better tomorrow and that there are things that you can do to improve your quality of life. Through careful planning and prioritization, you can learn to conserve your energy resources and use them most efficiently. This way, you can avoid exhaustion, better manage your chronic pain, and lead a fulfilling life.

PLANNING YOUR DAY

As a person with this chronic pain condition, you know that living with fibromyalgia involves navigating unpredictable energy levels. You can admit that you cannot do certain tasks at a given time; once you feel stronger, you can deal with them. Remember that by implementing some strategies and making careful choices, planning a day that maximizes energy levels and minimizes feelings of fatigue is possible.

Here are some insights and strategies to consider when you are planning your day:

1. **Prioritize and set realistic goals:** Start by identifying the day's most important tasks or activities. Consider your energy levels and choose tasks that align with your priorities. Keep your goals realistic and focus on what can be accomplished with your available energy.

2. **Practice pacing:** Pacing is a key strategy for managing energy levels. Break down your activities into smaller, manageable tasks and intersperse them with rest periods. Pace yourself, alternating between more demanding and lighter tasks to avoid overexertion.

3. **Listen to your body:** Pay close attention to your body's cues and signals. If you start feeling fatigued or experiencing pain, take a break and allow yourself time to rest and recharge. Pushing through the fatigue can lead to worsening symptoms and prolonged recovery time.

4. **Time management:** It can be helpful to allocate specific time slots for tasks and activities. It's important to establish and maintain a consistent daily routine. This can help regulate your energy levels and reduce decision fatigue.

5. **Delegate and ask for help:** Recognize that you don't have to do everything alone. Delegate tasks to family members and friends, or consider hiring assistance for certain activities. Asking for help can conserve your energy and prevent overwhelming fatigue.

6. **Optimize your environment:** Create a supportive environment that minimizes physical and mental strain. Organize your living and working spaces to reduce the need for excessive physical effort. Create a calm and comfortable setting that promotes relaxation and minimizes stress.

7. **Practice stress management:** Stress can exacerbate fatigue and other symptoms. It is important to incorporate different stress management techniques like deep breathing, meditation, mindfulness, or gentle exercises into your daily routine. Implementing these practices can be an effective way to lower your stress levels and save your energy.

8. **Maintain a healthy lifestyle:** Prioritize healthy habits such as getting regular quality sleep, eating a balanced diet, and staying hydrated. Good nutrition and proper rest can support your overall energy levels and well-being.

9. **Connect with support networks:** Seek support from others who understand and can empathize with your experience. Joining support groups or online communities can provide valuable emotional support, practical advice, and a sense of belonging.

10. **Adjust expectations and practice self-compassion:** It is important to recognize that living with fibromyalgia means that you will be facing limitations. Adjust your expectations and be kind to yourself. Celebrate your small achievements and practice self-compassion, acknowledging that you are doing your best in managing your condition.

Remember, everyone's experience with fibromyalgia is unique, and what works for one person may not work for another. Finding the best strategies that work best for you may take time, trial, and error. Be patient, stay flexible, and continue to learn and adapt as you navigate your journey with fibromyalgia.

UNDERSTAND YOUR ENERGY PATTERNS

Understanding your energy patterns is important for managing your productivity and well-being. Here are some additional details:

1. Everyone has natural peaks and troughs of energy throughout the day. These are periods when you feel more alert, focused, and energetic, as well as times when fatigue and low energy levels are more pronounced. These patterns can vary from person to person and can be especially noticeable for people with fibromyalgia.
2. You can keep an energy diary for a week to better understand your energy patterns. This involves writing down specific times when you experience your highest energy levels and when fatigue hits the hardest. You can record this information in a journal, on your phone, or using any other convenient method.
3. By maintaining an energy diary, you can start identifying your personal energy windows. These are the periods of the day when you have the most energy and are most capable of engaging in tasks requiring

higher concentration and focus. Recognizing these windows allows you to plan your activities accordingly and maximize your productivity during these times.

4. Additionally, noting when fatigue is most intense can help you to identify potential triggers or factors contributing to your energy depletion. This information can be valuable in making lifestyle adjustments, such as managing your activities, incorporating rest breaks, or seeking medical advice if needed.

Prioritize tasks

Fibromyalgia warriors need to remember to be kind to and patient with themselves. It is also important for a fibromyalgia warrior to remember that even people who are perfectly "healthy" often struggle to prioritize tasks.

Prioritizing tasks is the act of organizing and arranging your tasks based on their importance, urgency, and energy requirements. Not all tasks are equal, and by prioritizing them effectively, you can make better use of your time and energy, increase productivity, and reduce stress.

By understanding the energy levels required for different tasks and aligning them with your periods of peak energy, you can optimize your workflow and efficiently manage your workload. This approach optimizes productivity by matching tasks to energy levels. Prioritizing tasks also helps you stay organized, make informed decisions about allocating your time, and achieve your goals more effectively.

By prioritizing tasks based on your energy levels, you can begin to optimize your productivity and manage your energy efficiently. Here's a breakdown of how to do it:

1. **Recognize task energy requirements:** Understand that different tasks have varying levels of mental or physical energy demands. Some tasks may require intense concentration, problem-solving, or physical exertion, while others may involve lighter, routine activities.

2. **Identify your energy peaks:** Refer to your energy diary to determine when you typically experience higher energy levels. These are the periods when you feel most alert, focused, and capable of tackling more demanding tasks more efficiently.

3. **Schedule demanding tasks:** Assign the mentally or physically demanding tasks to your identified energy peaks. During these periods, your energy reserves are at their highest, allowing you to tackle complex or challenging tasks more effectively.

4. **Save less demanding tasks:** Reserve tasks that require less mental or physical energy for the times when you're typically more fatigued. These can include more routine and administrative activities or be broken down into smaller steps. Doing this allows you to still progress on tasks during periods of lower energy without feeling overwhelmed.

5. **Take breaks:** Remember to incorporate regular breaks throughout your day, regardless of task demands. These breaks allow you to recharge and prevent fatigue from

building up, ensuring sustained productivity and well-being.

By aligning task prioritization with your energy levels, you can optimize your work schedule and efficiently use your available energy resources. This approach will help you to minimize fatigue, increase productivity, and maintain a healthier balance between work and rest.

Pace yourself

Pacing yourself is an important strategy for managing your energy levels, avoiding burnout, and maintaining a consistent level of productivity throughout the day. Continuously pushing through fatigue can lead to physical and mental exhaustion, resulting in crashes or exacerbated symptoms.

By breaking tasks into manageable chunks and interspersing them with short breaks, you can prevent overexertion and maintain a more sustainable energy level. Pacing yourself helps to optimize your productivity, reduce the risk of burnout, and promote a healthier balance between work and rest. By prioritizing self-care and listening to your body's needs, you can achieve a more sustainable and effective approach to managing your daily activities.

Pacing yourself is essential for managing your energy levels and avoiding burnout. Here are some key points to keep in mind:

1. **Recognize the consequences of pushing through fatigue:** Ignoring signs of fatigue and overexerting yourself can have negative consequences, such as

increased symptoms, decreased productivity, and heightened exhaustion. It's important to listen to your body and prioritize self-care.

2. **Break tasks into manageable chunks:** Instead of trying to complete a task in one sitting, divide it into smaller, more manageable parts. This allows you to focus on one part at a time, reducing your risk of mental and physical strain.

3. **Intersperse tasks with short breaks:** Take regular breaks between tasks or after completing each chunk. Use this time to rest, relax, and recharge. Even short breaks can help refresh your mind and prevent excessive fatigue.

4. **Maintain a consistent energy level:** By pacing yourself and taking breaks, you can maintain a more consistent energy level throughout the day. This helps to prevent overexertion and minimizes the likelihood of experiencing extreme highs and lows in energy.

Remember, pacing yourself is not a sign of weakness but rather a strategic approach to optimize your energy and well-being. By giving yourself the necessary breaks and breaking tasks into manageable chunks, you can work more efficiently, reduce the risk of crashes, and maintain a healthier balance in managing your daily activities.

Mind Your Mental Energy

Taking care of your mental energy is essential for maintaining focus, productivity, and overall well-being. Here are some key points to remember:

1. **Recognize the impact of mental fatigue:** Mental fatigue can significantly impact your ability to concentrate, make good decisions, and perform tasks effectively. Acknowledging and addressing mental exhaustion is important, just as you would with physical fatigue.

2. **Take short mental breaks:** Incorporate regular mental breaks into your day. These breaks can be as simple as taking a few moments to practice deep breathing exercises, which can help relax your mind and reduce stress. Alternatively, you can listen to calming music or step outside to get fresh air and rejuvenate your mental energy.

3. **Find activities that recharge your mind:** Explore different activities that help you relax and recharge mentally. This could include engaging in mindfulness exercises, practicing meditation or yoga, reading a book, or pursuing a hobby you enjoy. These activities can refresh your mental state and increase your focus and productivity.

By prioritizing your mental energy and taking regular breaks to recharge, you can prevent mental exhaustion, maintain a clearer and more focused mindset, and enhance your ability to tackle tasks effectively. It's important to listen to your mind's needs and incorporate activities that promote mental well-being into your daily routine.

Prepare for Tomorrow, But Stay Flexible

Striking a balance between preparation and flexibility is important when managing your tasks and daily routine. Here are some key points to consider:

1. **Plan ahead to reduce decision fatigue:** Ending your day with a plan for the next day can help alleviate morning decision fatigue. Taking a few minutes each evening to outline your priorities allows you to start each morning with clarity and purpose, increasing your productivity and reducing stress.

2. **Remain adaptable due to the unpredictability of fibromyalgia:** It is important to acknowledge that fibromyalgia can be unpredictable, and symptoms may vary from day to day. Despite the best planning, you may face challenges and unforeseen setbacks. Additionally, it is important to become comfortable with being flexible and adjusting your plans to accommodate your fluctuating energy levels.

3. **Listen to your body and give yourself grace:** If you are having a particularly challenging day, it is important to listen to your body and prioritize self-care. Adjusting your plans or activities is perfectly alright and should not be seen as a failure. Giving yourself grace and understanding allows you to focus on your well-being, modify, and ensure long-term productivity and self-care.

By preparing for the next day while maintaining flexibility, you can balance structure and adaptability. This approach helps you optimize your productivity, manage the unpredictability of fibromyalgia, and prioritize self-care effectively. Remember to be kind to yourself and embrace the necessary changes to create a routine that works best for you.

Navigating Nightly Rest with Fibromyalgia

Sleep is vital to your well-being, and it is particularly crucial if you have fibromyalgia. The relationship between fibromyalgia and sleep is complex, with various sleep disorders often accompanying the condition. Understanding how fibromyalgia affects sleep and implementing strategies to improve sleep quality can significantly enhance daily functioning and quality of life.

Fibromyalgia can disrupt sleep in several ways, including:

1. **Insomnia:** Insomnia, characterized by difficulty falling asleep or staying asleep, is commonly experienced by people with fibromyalgia. Pain, discomfort, anxiety, and other symptoms can make it challenging to achieve restful sleep.
2. **Sleep Apnea:** Sleep apnea, a disorder where breathing repeatedly stops and starts during sleep, is prevalent in fibromyalgia warriors. Sleep apnea can further disrupt sleep patterns, contributing to fatigue and daytime sleepiness.
3. **Restless Legs Syndrome:** Restless Legs Syndrome (RLS) causes uncomfortable sensations in your legs, which is often accompanied by an irresistible urge to

move them. RLS can make it difficult to find a comfortable position and fall asleep.

Given the importance of sleep for managing fibromyalgia symptoms, here are some tips that you can use to improve your sleep quality:

- Avoid stimulants and alcohol late in the day to promote better sleep quality.
- Create a sleep-friendly environment by sleeping in a dark and quiet room. Consider using earplugs, eye masks, or white noise machines if needed.
- Establish a relaxing pre-sleep routine, such as taking a warm bath or shower before bed.
- Minimize daytime napping to avoid disrupting the sleep-wake cycle. If necessary, limit naps to short and early afternoon durations.
- Engage in light stretches or gentle exercises before bedtime every night to promote relaxation and improve sleep quality.
- Experiment with different body positions and use body pillows to find the most comfortable and supportive position for sleep.
- Consider incorporating relaxing music into your nighttime routine to create a peaceful atmosphere.
- Discuss the option of sleep medications with your healthcare provider if necessary.
- Enjoy a good book before bed to unwind and prepare your mind for sleep.

- Instead of tossing and turning in bed when you cannot sleep, get up and do something that relaxes you until you feel sleepy again.
- Taking time off work when needed to prioritize rest and self-care is important for managing fibromyalgia symptoms.
- Embrace an active and healthy lifestyle, including regular exercise, a healthy balanced diet, and stress management techniques, as they can positively impact sleep quality.

Remember, managing fibromyalgia and improving sleep quality is a journey that may require individualized approaches. It's important to work with healthcare professionals to find the best strategies for your specific needs. Prioritizing restful sleep is key in managing your fibromyalgia symptoms and promoting overall well-being.

In the chapter *The Power of Pause*, we explored the significance of taking breaks and allowing yourself moments of rest and rejuvenation. By understanding the importance of pacing yourself, minding your mental and physical energy, and prioritizing sleep, you can optimize your productivity and well-being. We discussed the transformative power of sleep and the relationship between fibromyalgia and sleep, acknowledging the various sleep disorders that often accompany the condition.

Strategies for improving sleep quality were also provided, such as avoiding stimulants, creating a sleep-friendly environment, engaging in relaxation techniques, and seeking medical guidance when necessary. By navigating nightly rest with fibromyalgia, you can enhance your overall lifestyle and effectively manage the challenges of the condition.

In the upcoming chapter, we will delve into the fascinating topic of the *Fibromyalgia-Food Connection*. We will explore how dietary choices and nutrition can influence fibromyalgia symptoms, energy levels, inflammation, and overall well-being. Understanding the role of food in managing fibromyalgia can empower you as a warrior to make informed decisions and create personalized dietary strategies to support your health. From identifying potential trigger foods to incorporating anti-inflammatory and nutrient-dense options, you will navigate the impact of food on fibromyalgia symptoms. Stay tuned to discover how a thoughtful approach to nutrition can contribute to a healthier, more balanced life with fibromyalgia.

4

THE FIBROMYALGIA-FOOD CONNECTION

P eople say, "You are what you eat." In the context of fibromyalgia, how might the foods we consume influence our symptoms, and how can we harness the power of nutrition to find relief?

The relationship between certain foods and fibromyalgia symptoms is quite intriguing. While many people's experiences can vary, some people with fibromyalgia find that certain foods can impact their symptoms. Commonly reported triggers include additives, preservatives, artificial sweeteners, and high-processed foods.

Moreover, some people have noted that a diet rich in fruits, vegetables, lean proteins, and whole grains might help alleviate symptoms. It is always a good idea to keep a food diary to track how different foods make you feel, as this can offer personalized insights into what works best for managing fibromyalgia symptoms.

This chapter explores the connection between diet and fibromyalgia symptoms. You will gain insights into how your dietary choices can impact your symptoms and discover practical strategies for personalized nutrition.

FOOD AND FIBROMYALGIA

When you are living with a condition like fibromyalgia, it is important that you aim to eat a well-rounded diet. According to a 2018 literature review, it is important for people with fibromyalgia to obtain the proper combination of nutrients. Diets that are abundant in antioxidants and provide sufficient nutrients, like vitamin B12, can contribute to alleviating symptoms.

A balanced diet should include the following:

- fresh fruits
- fresh vegetables
- healthy fats
- lean protein, like chicken or fish
- low-fat dairy
- whole grains

Avoid foods with low nutritional value, as they are more likely to harm your health. This includes excessive amounts of saturated fats and anything fried or processed. Also, remember to limit the amount of salt and sugar you consume in your diet.

Eat for Energy

Consuming specific foods can provide you with additional energy to help you navigate your day. To regulate the absorption of carbohydrates, try pairing them with protein or healthy fats. Opt for fresh, whole foods that are very rich in fiber and low in added sugars, like:

- avocado
- beans
- broccoli
- dark leafy greens
- nuts
- oatmeal
- seeds
- tofu

Avoid sweets, as they only provide a quick sugar boost. Your body will quickly burn through them, leading to a subsequent crash or the immediate loss of that high-energy feeling.

Go Vegetarian

Several older studies have examined the impact of specific diets on fibromyalgia. In a small study conducted in 2000, it was concluded that following a raw and vegan diet may provide relief from symptoms like joint stiffness and poor sleep.

Another study, published in BMC Complementary and Alternative Medicine 2001, found that people who primarily consumed raw and vegetarian foods, such as salads, carrot juice, nuts, and fruits, experienced reduced pain.

More recent research has also highlighted the benefits of a raw and vegetarian diet (Nadal-Nicolás et al., 2021). A literature review conducted in 2019 reported that people who followed this type of diet for a few months observed improvements in various parameters.

- emotional health
- morning stiffness
- pain
- sleep quality

While plant-based diets are generally healthy and rich in antioxidants, raw food diets are highly restrictive and may not be suitable for everyone.

Avoid Foods That Trigger Symptoms

While there is no single fibromyalgia diet, research indicates that certain ingredients or foods may cause additional problems for some people with fibromyalgia (Stephens, 2022). Certain types of foods can have an impact on how you feel. Try to keep a detailed food diary to help you identify which foods may trigger or improve your symptoms.

Let us have a look at foods that most commonly trigger symptoms in people with fibromyalgia, including:

- excitotoxins
- fermentable oligosaccharide, disaccharide, monosaccharide, and polyols
- gluten

Fermentable Oligosaccharide, Disaccharide, Monosaccharide, and Polyols (FODMAPs)

A 2017 study found that some fibromyalgia warriors had improved symptoms and quality of life when they followed a low-FODMAP diet. The good news is that people following this diet also lose weight. FODMAPs are carbohydrates fermented by gut bacteria in the digestive tract. They may promote symptoms in some people.

Foods that are high in FODMAPs include:

- barley and rye
- beans
- bread
- cruciferous vegetables like broccoli, Brussels sprouts, and cauliflower
- dairy products
- fruits such as apples, peaches, and pears
- pasta

Gluten

A 2014 study found that adhering to a gluten-free diet can help improve pain and quality-of-life indicators in people with fibromyalgia who tested negative for celiac disease, indicating that non-celiac gluten sensitivity may be an underlying cause.

Gluten can be found in various foods, including:

- Barley: Malt, malt vinegar, and some types of beer.
- Rye: Rye bread, rye beer, and certain cereals.
- Some oats: Sometimes, oats can be cross-contaminated with gluten-containing grains during processing.
- Wheat-based products: Bread, pasta, couscous, crackers, and baked goods.

It is also important to remember that many processed foods might contain gluten as an additive, so if you specifically avoid it, you should check the labels.

Excitotoxins

Excitotoxins like MSG and aspartame stimulate the tongue's taste receptors. Eliminating them may help relieve pain symptoms in people with fibromyalgia and IBS. However, larger studies are needed to fully understand the impact of excitotoxins on the human body.

Foods that might contain Excitotoxins include:

- certain flavored chips
- certain restaurant foods

- certain sauces or dressings
- processed meats
- some soups

MAINTAINING A MODERATE WEIGHT

Consuming a healthy diet can help you manage weight and alleviate fibromyalgia symptoms. A 2012 study showed that losing weight can improve the quality of life for people who are living with fibromyalgia (Dellwo, 2014). Similarly, a 2019 literature review found that losing weight and following a low-calorie diet can reduce pain and inflammation, leading to a better quality of life.

There are no two ways about it that managing your weight when you are living with fibromyalgia can be tough. It requires a delicate balance, especially given the challenges of pain and fatigue. Here are some tips that might help you:

1. **Balanced Diet:** Focus on a well-rounded diet. Avoid processed foods and excess sugar.
2. **Portion Control:** Pay attention to portion sizes to maintain calorie intake. Smaller, frequent meals might be easier to manage than larger ones.
3. **Stay Active:** While it might be challenging, gentle exercise can help you manage your weight. Always consult a healthcare provider or physical therapist to find suitable exercises for your condition.

4. **Mindful Movement:** Incorporate movement into your routine. Short bursts of activity throughout the day, like stretching or light house chores, can add up.

5. **Stress Management:** Stress can exacerbate fibromyalgia symptoms. Techniques like meditation, deep breathing, or hobbies that relax you can help manage stress levels, potentially impacting weight.

6. **Medication Management:** Work closely with your healthcare provider to manage your medications, as some might affect weight.

7. **Quality Sleep:** Aim for good sleep hygiene. Quality sleep can impact weight management and overall health.

Remember, it is essential to approach weight management in a way that does not exacerbate your fibromyalgia symptoms. Consulting with healthcare professionals specializing in fibromyalgia and nutrition could provide tailored advice for your situation.

NATURAL FIBROMYALGIA REMEDIES

Some people work hard to improve their fibromyalgia symptoms with herbal remedies and dietary supplements. Unfortunately, there is not much research to show that these supplements do work. While there are a few studies done, they did not find much improvement in fibromyalgia symptoms.

If you are in search of natural remedies to help you manage your fibromyalgia symptoms, please do so with great caution.

It is not easy to find people online selling miracle cures for fibromyalgia which do not work. Please be vigilant so that you do not spend your hard-earned money on empty promises of miracle cures to offer you relief from your symptoms.

Researchers are investigating possible connections between nutritional deficiencies and fibromyalgia symptoms. However, a 2017 literature review found no evidence of vitamin and mineral deficiencies affecting fibromyalgia.

Research suggests a link between fibromyalgia pain and low levels of nutrients like magnesium, calcium, and vitamin D. However, more studies are needed to confirm this.

Animal products, such as yogurt and salmon, are excellent sources of calcium and vitamin D. People following vegan or vegetarian diets must remember to plan carefully to get these nutrients into their diets. If you follow a meat-free diet, make sure to include almonds, mushrooms, tofu, and fortified foods in your meals to ensure you are getting adequate nutrition.

Additionally, taking time to enjoy a warm bath with Epsom salts a few times a week can help you relieve fibromyalgia symptoms such as pain.

The Bottom Line

While there is no cure for fibromyalgia, and limited research exists on the impact of diet on the disease, modifying your diet may help alleviate some of your symptoms. Following a diet with plenty of vegetables and fruits is recommended. Additionally, pay attention to which foods appear to worsen your symptoms.

Promising outcomes have been observed in clinical trials that involved supplementing with vitamin D, magnesium, iron, and probiotics. In terms of dietary approaches, the use of olive oil, incorporating ancient grains into the diet, adopting low-calorie diets, following the low FODMAPs diet, gluten-free diet, monosodium glutamate and aspartame-free diet, vegetarian diets, and the Mediterranean diet have all shown effectiveness in alleviating FM symptoms.

THE LINK BETWEEN GUT HEALTH AND FIBROMYALGIA

While the exact cause of fibromyalgia is currently unknown, recent research suggests that there may be a link between gut health and the development and management of fibromyalgia symptoms.

The gut microbiome, comprising trillions of microorganisms in your digestive system, plays an important role in maintaining overall health and well-being. Studies have shown that people living with fibromyalgia have an altered gut microbiome with a lower amount of helpful bacteria and a higher amount of harmful bacteria.(Franz Martín et al., 2023).

A balanced gut microbiome is vital for proper immune function, digestion, and the production of neurotransmitters that regulate mood and pain perception. When your gut microbiome is imbalanced, it may lead to increased inflammation, compromised immune function, and heightened pain sensitivity, all of which are common features of fibromyalgia.

Managing fibromyalgia symptoms requires a multifaceted approach, and improving gut health is becoming an important aspect of treatment. Adopting a diet rich in fiber, prebiotics, and probiotics can help nourish the beneficial bacteria in the gut and restore balance. Additionally, certain dietary modifications, such as reducing processed foods, sugar, and artificial additives, may alleviate symptoms and promote a healthier gut environment.

Furthermore, addressing gut health through lifestyle changes and, when necessary, supplementation may help reduce inflammation, manage pain, and improve the overall well-being of people with fibromyalgia.

The link between gut health and fibromyalgia highlights how important a balanced gut microbiome in overall well-being and symptom management is. By nourishing the gut with a healthy diet and adopting lifestyle strategies that support gut health, individuals with fibromyalgia may experience improvements in their symptoms and overall quality of life.

Add Nutritiotnal Friends and Foes

Here are some guidelines for choosing foods for fibromyalgia:

- **It is best to steer clear of foods that have added glutamate in them:** Glutamate is an excitatory neurotransmitter that can worsen symptoms in some people with fibromyalgia. Foods to avoid include processed meats, snacks, and some flavor enhancers.

- **Choose whole foods instead of processed ones**: Rather than processed foods, opt for whole, nutritious foods like fruits, vegetables, whole grains, lean proteins, and healthy fats. These foods provide essential nutrients and are often lower in additives that can trigger symptoms.
- **Try the DASH or Mediterranean eating plan**. DASH and Mediterranean diets emphasize whole foods, fruits, veggies, lean proteins, and healthy fats. These diets are linked to lower risk of chronic diseases and may alleviate fibromyalgia symptoms.
- **Avoid cured meats**: Cured meats, such as bacon, ham, and sausages, often contain additives and preservatives that can trigger symptoms in some individuals. Opt for fresh, lean meats or plant-based protein sources instead.
- **Eat cold-water fish and fortified foods for Vitamin D**: It has been shown that a lack of Vitamin D increases pain sensitivity. Add fatty fish like salmon and fortified foods like milk and cereals to ensure enough Vitamin D intake.
- **Choose dark, leafy greens, nuts, and seeds for magnesium**. Magnesium helps with muscle relaxation and nerve function, which may benefit people living with fibromyalgia. Add spinach, kale, almonds, and sunflower seeds to your diet.
- **Add in fish, flaxseed, and chia for Omega-3 fatty acids**: Omega-3 fatty acids, known for their anti-

inflammatory properties, may help reduce pain and inflammation. Include sources like fatty fish (salmon, mackerel), flaxseeds, and chia seeds in your meals.

- **Include antioxidants in your meals**: Antioxidants can help reduce oxidative stress and inflammation. Consume various fruits and vegetables, particularly those rich in vibrant colors like berries, cherries, spinach, and bell peppers.
- **Read the labels on packaged foods**: Pay attention to ingredient lists and nutritional information on packaged foods. Avoid products that contain additives, preservatives, high levels of sodium, or artificial ingredients that may trigger symptoms.
- **Avoid artificial sweeteners and limit sugars**: Some people with fibromyalgia may experience exacerbated symptoms after consuming artificial sweeteners and excessive amounts of sugar. Opt for natural sweeteners in moderation, or choose naturally sweetened foods.

Foods Commonly Beneficial For People With Fibromyalgia

Here is a comprehensive list of foods commonly considered beneficial for people with fibromyalgia, as well as those that might exacerbate symptoms:

Foods beneficial for fibromyalgia:

- **Fruits:** Berries (such as blueberries, strawberries, and raspberries), cherries, oranges, pineapple, and mangoes.
- **Vegetables:** Leafy greens, broccoli, Brussels sprouts, cauliflower, bell peppers, and sweet potatoes.
- **Whole grains:** Quinoa, brown rice, oats, whole wheat bread, and whole grain pasta.
- **Lean proteins:** Skinless poultry, fish (such as salmon, mackerel, and trout), tofu, beans, and lentils.
- **Healthy fats:** Avocado, olive oil, nuts (such as almonds, walnuts, and pistachios), and seeds (such as flaxseeds and chia seeds).
- **Low-fat dairy or Dairy Alternatives:** Greek yogurt, almond milk, and fortified plant-based milk.
- **Omega-3 Fatty Acids:** Fatty fish, flaxseeds, chia seeds, and walnuts.
- **Vitamin D Sources:** Cold-water fish (such as salmon and mackerel), fortified dairy or plant-based milk, and sunlight exposure.
- **Magnesium-rich foods:** Dark leafy greens, nuts, seeds, and legumes.
- **Antioxidant-rich foods include berries** (such as blueberries and strawberries), cherries, dark chocolate (in moderation), spinach, kale, and colorful fruits and vegetables.
- **Herbal teas:** Chamomile, ginger, turmeric, and peppermint tea can be soothing.

Foods to Limit or Avoid that might trigger your Fibromyalgia symptoms:

- **Processed foods:** These include packaged snacks, fast food, frozen meals, pre-packaged sauces, and instant noodles, as they often contain additives and preservatives that may trigger symptoms.
- **Artificial sweeteners:** Aspartame, sucralose, saccharin, and other artificial sweeteners are found in diet sodas, sugar-free products, and some low-sugar or diabetic-friendly foods. They may exacerbate symptoms in some people.
- **Caffeine:** While moderate amounts of caffeine can provide temporary energy, excessive consumption (found in coffee, energy drinks, and some sodas) may disrupt sleep patterns and contribute to muscle tension and pain.
- **High-sugar foods:** Limit foods high in added sugars, such as sugary desserts, candies, pastries, and sweetened beverages.
- **High-fat and fried foods** include fatty cuts of meat, deep-fried foods, and high-fat dairy products like full-fat cheese and butter.
- **Excessive sodium:** Limit foods high in sodium, like processed meats, canned soups, and fast food, as they may contribute to inflammation and water retention.

Remember, different people's responses to food can vary, so it is important to pay attention to your body's specific reactions and consult a healthcare professional or registered dietitian for personalized advice.

THE ROLE OF HYDRATION

Staying hydrated is indeed important for managing fibromyalgia symptoms. Here is why hydration is crucial and how it can help:

1. **Enhanced digestion**: People with fibromyalgia often experience constipation. Drinking adequate water promotes regular bowel movements, prevents constipation, and supports proper digestion.
2. **Improved energy levels**: Fatigue is a common symptom of fibromyalgia. When you are dehydrated, you may experience low energy and decreased cognitive function. Drinking enough water helps optimize energy levels and mental clarity.
3. **Joint and muscle health**: Hydration aids in lubricating your joints and delivering nutrients to the muscles. It may help alleviate stiffness, improve flexibility, and reduce muscle cramps and spasms often associated with fibromyalgia.
4. **Pain relief**: Dehydration can contribute to increased pain perception and sensitivity. By maintaining proper hydration, you can reduce the intensity of fibromyalgia pain.
5. **Temperature regulation**: Fibromyalgia can impact the body's thermoregulation, making people more sensitive to temperature changes. Staying hydrated assists in

maintaining normal body temperature, which can help manage temperature-related symptoms.

To ensure proper hydration for fibromyalgia management, keep the following in mind:

- **Include hydrating foods**: To supplement hydration, incorporate foods with high water content, such as fruits (watermelon, citrus fruits), vegetables (cucumbers, lettuce), and soups.
- **Limit dehydrating beverages**: Avoid excessive consumption of caffeinated and alcoholic, as they can contribute to dehydration. These drinks have diuretic effects, causing increased urination and potential fluid loss.
- **Monitor urine color**: It is important to pay attention to the color of your urine. Pale or light yellow urine indicates proper hydration, while darker urine suggests dehydration.
- **Sip throughout the day**: To stay hydrated, sip water regularly throughout the day rather than consuming large amounts all at once.
- **Water intake**: Aim to drink at least 8 cups (64 ounces) of water daily. Adjust your intake based on climate, activity level, and your needs.

Remember, your hydration needs may vary, so listen to your body's signals and adjust your water intake accordingly. It is always good to consult a healthcare professional for personalized advice on hydration and fibromyalgia management.

In this chapter, we explored the link between fibromyalgia and food, emphasizing the importance of making informed choices to support symptom management and overall well-being. We discussed beneficial foods for fibromyalgia, such as fruits, vegetables, whole grains, lean proteins, healthy fats, and specific nutrients like omega-3 fatty acids, magnesium, and antioxidants. We also highlighted the need to avoid certain foods, including processed products, artificial sweeteners, high-sugar foods, and excessive sodium.

Building upon the understanding of the fibromyalgia-food connection, the next chapter delves into the role of movement as medicine in managing fibromyalgia symptoms. We will explore the benefits of exercise, stretches, and other physical activities in improving muscle strength, flexibility, and overall physical and mental well-being. Stay tuned to discover how movement can be a logical continuation in your journey towards managing fibromyalgia effectively.

5

MOVEMENT AS MEDICINE

Many people who are suffering from chronic musculoskeletal (MSK) pain find it easier to avoid movement that is causing pain. However, exercise helps the brain and body manage pain and is often the best way to help ease the pain.

Movement as medicine refers to the idea that physical activity and exercise are vital in promoting overall health and well-being. This concept emphasizes the profound benefits of incorporating movement, exercise, and physical activity as a fundamental part of maintaining a healthy lifestyle.

When approached as a form of medicine, exercise has multifaceted advantages beyond just physical fitness. It has a powerful impact on mental health and emotional well-being and even plays a role in preventing various chronic diseases. This chapter will explore ways that you can use movement as medicine.

EXERCISE AND FIBROMYALGIA MANAGEMENT

Fibromyalgia affects millions of people worldwide, and while there is no cure currently, managing your symptoms is important to improving your quality of life. One of the most effective ways to manage the symptoms of fibromyalgia is through regular exercise.

Even though engaging in physical activity may seem counterintuitive when you are living with chronic pain and fatigue, exercise really can be a powerful tool in managing the condition. However, when you have fibromyalgia, it is important to approach any exercise correctly and to seek advice from a healthcare professional or an exercise specialist to develop an exercise plan that is tailored to your abilities and limitations.

Regular exercise, when approached correctly, can help manage fibromyalgia symptoms. Exercise can offer you numerous benefits; here are some of the key advantages:

1. **Pain Management:** Regular exercise can help reduce your pain levels. It promotes the release of endorphins, which are natural pain-relieving chemicals in your body. Regular exercise can be beneficial in improving flexibility and muscle strength, which may help to reduce muscle soreness and stiffness. Additionally, exercise can also improve overall physical fitness and well-being.

2. **Improved Sleep:** Engaging in physical activity can greatly enhance your quality of sleep when you have fibromyalgia. Regular exercise also helps regulate your

sleep-wake cycle and promotes deeper and more restful sleep, reducing fatigue and restoring energy levels.

3. **Increased Energy Levels:** Although fibromyalgia often causes fatigue, exercise can actually increase your energy levels. Physical activity also improves your cardiovascular fitness and stimulates the production of energy-boosting hormones, ultimately reducing feelings of fatigue and enhancing overall vitality.

4. **Mental Well-being:** Regular exercise has several benefits for your mental health. Triggering the release of endorphins can help improve mood, reducing anxiety, depression, and stress, thus promoting overall mental well-being. Exercise can also provide a sense of accomplishment and empowerment, which can boost your self-esteem and confidence.

5. **Improved Functionality:** Regular exercise can also improve your physical functionality, enabling you to perform your daily tasks more easily. It will enhance your muscle strength, flexibility, and endurance, improving mobility, balance, and coordination.

6. **Enhanced Overall Health:** Exercise offers various health benefits beyond just fibromyalgia management. It can help improve your overall health by maintaining a healthy weight, and reduce the risk of chronic diseases such as diabetes and heart disease, and enhancing cardiovascular health.

Incorporating regular exercise and movement into your daily life can significantly contribute to a healthier, more balanced lifestyle, fostering long-term physical and mental well-being.

The key is finding activities that you can genuinely enjoy and sustain so that you can reap the myriad benefits of movement as medicine.

PROVEN EXERCISES TO HELP EASE FIBROMYALGIA PAIN

Stating that living with fibromyalgia can be tough is an understatement, but with courage, you can. It affects your muscles, ligaments, and joints, causing widespread chronic pain that can make exercising seem like a real challenge. Along with that, fatigue, sleep issues, and trouble focusing can really take a toll.

Now, while medications can help alleviate the symptoms, the American College of Rheumatology actually suggests including exercise alongside any prescribed medicine. It is all about finding gentle, tailored exercises that work for you and your body to enhance your overall well-being.

By now you understand that scientists are still unravelling the mysteries that lie behind the triggers of fibromyalgia. So, you might be wondering how exactly exercise can help you with fibromyalgia. While dealing with persistent muscle pain might make you feel less inclined to be as active as you would want to be, you absolutely need to summon up every ounce of courage in your being and get some exercise.

You might be concerned that exercising could make your pain symptoms worse, and that is completely reasonable. However, studies indicate that over time, exercise could actually help alleviate the symptoms. There are some potential perks to exercising with fibromyalgia, such as:

- Feeling less tired: Exercise could help reduce fatigue and improve the quality of your sleep if you are dealing with fibromyalgia.
- Reduced discomfort: It might seem counterintuitive to exercise with musculoskeletal pain, but it can actually lessen chronic pain associated with fibromyalgia.
- Boosted physical well-being: Regular exercise can enhance heart health, muscle strength, and flexibility. Even people with fibromyalgia can benefit from this.
- Happier vibes: Those with fibromyalgia face a higher risk of depression, but the good news is that exercise is a great mood booster. Setting aside time for workouts could help alleviate symptoms of depression and anxiety.
- Sharper mind: Staying active can assist people with fibromyalgia in improving their working memory and overall cognitive function.

EXERCISE FOR FIBROMYALGIA

Although there is no one-size-fits-all exercise plan for fibromyalgia, research indicates that aerobic workouts and strength training can be beneficial in managing the condition. Additionally, there is limited yet encouraging evidence that mind-body practices might offer some help, too.

As a fibromyalgia warrior, there are several different types of exercises that can help you live your best life. It is important to choose exercises that suit your unique preferences and abilities. Please remember that an exercise plan for fibromyalgia should be low-impact. Always listen to your body and pace yourself during exercise. Start by slowly and gradually increase the intensity and duration of your workouts as tolerated.

Here are some common types of exercises that are often recommended for fibromyalgia management:

Aerobics

Low-Impact Aerobic Exercises like walking, swimming, cycling, or using an elliptical machine can improve cardiovascular fitness without putting excessive strain on the joints. Remember to start with gentle exercises and gradually increase intensity and duration over time.

Aerobic exercise can work wonders for easing fibromyalgia pain, reducing stiffness, and enhancing overall function. Various types of aerobic activities can be really effective, such as:

Walking

Walking can also be an incredibly beneficial form of exercise when you are living with fibromyalgia. It is a fantastic, low-impact exercise, especially if you are just starting out with an exercise regime. You can gradually boost the intensity by trying Nordic walking, which engages upper and lower body muscles.

Here is exactly how walking can help you:

- Boosts Mental Well-being: In addition to the physical benefits, walking can also positively affect your mental well-being. Engaging in outdoor activities can provide stress relief, alleviate pain, and foster social connections. Exercise and fresh air can help relieve symptoms of depression and anxiety associated with fibromyalgia.
- Builds Strength and Flexibility: Walking involves activating various muscle groups, including the legs, hips, and the core. Over time, regular walking can help strengthen these muscles, increase flexibility, and improve your overall physical function. This can be particularly beneficial if you experience muscle weakness or stiffness.
- Enhances Sleep Quality: Regular exercise, including walking, will improve sleep quality.Incorporating a daily walking routine can improve sleep patterns and promote restful sleep.
- Improves Circulation: Walking also enhances blood circulation throughout your body, promoting the delivery of oxygen and nutrients to the muscles and tissues. Improved circulation can help reduce your pain and stiffness and also aid in the removal of waste products from the muscles.
- Increases Endurance: Regular walking helps to gradually improve your cardiovascular endurance over time. This can be particularly helpful if you often experience fatigue and reduced stamina. By increasing

your endurance, walking can help improve your overall energy levels and reduce fatigue.

- Low-Impact Exercise: Walking is a good low-impact exercise that does not excessively strain your joints and muscles. This makes it an ideal choice, as it helps to minimize your risk of injury or flare-ups.
- Releases Endorphins: Engaging in moderate aerobic exercise, like brisk walking, stimulates the release of endorphins – your body's natural painkillers and mood boosters. This can help reduce pain perception, improve your mood, and promote a sense of well-being.

Water Aerobics

Taking your exercise routine to the water offers numerous benefits. The water's natural resistance can help increase muscle strength and flexibility while offering a low-impact workout. The therapeutic potential of water-based exercises includes:

- Buoyancy is key: Water provides a supportive environment that significantly reduces the impact on your joints. When engaging in exercises like stationary cycling or dancing in water, the natural buoyancy lessens strain on your joints, making it an excellent choice for people with joint pain or limited mobility.
- Mind-Body Harmony: For mind-body exercises like yoga and tai chi, water can be a serene setting to enhance these practices. The fluidity of water complements the flow and balance required for these

exercises, adding an extra element of tranquility and focus to your sessions.

- Resistance for Strength: The resistance from the water adds a whole new dimension to your workout. Dancing or engaging in strength training exercises in water offers a gentle yet effective way to strengthen your muscles. The water's resistance provides a constant challenge, aiding in strengthening your muscles. Water provides a constant challenge, helping muscle strengthening without the heavy strain often experienced with traditional exercises.
- Stretch and Relax: Stretching in water allows for a broader range of motion. The reduced pressure on your muscles encourages deeper stretches while minimizing the risk of injury.

Water-based exercises truly offer a holistic approach to wellness, catering to various fitness levels and health conditions. The environment is physically and mentally therapeutic, giving you a serene setting for your workout routines.

Cycling

Cycling is another excellent, low-impact option. If you are struggling with balance issues, then a stationary bike will reduce the risk of falls compared to outdoor cycling. Here's how cycling can help you:

- Cardiovascular Health: Cycling is an aerobic exercise that gets your heart rate up, improving cardiovascular health. Regular cycling can help improve blood circulation, increase lung capacity, and enhance overall cardiovascular endurance. This can help combat feelings of fatigue and improve overall energy levels.

- Joint Mobility: Cycling helps to promote joint mobility and range of motion, particularly in your hips, knees, and ankles. This can help increase flexibility and reduce stiffness, which can be particularly beneficial if you often experience joint pain and limited mobility.
- Low-Impact Exercise: Cycling is a low-impact exercise that minimizes the risk of injury.
- Mood Enhancement: Engaging in regular exercise, including cycling, promotes the release of endorphins. Cycling can help reduce depression, stress, and anxiety symptoms. It can also serve as a form of healthy distraction from pain and provide you with a sense of accomplishment and well-being.
- Muscle Strength: Cycling involves activating various muscle groups, like the legs, hips, and glutes. Regular cycling can help strengthen these muscles, which is beneficial if you experience muscle weakness or fatigue. Stronger muscles can support better joint stability and improve your overall physical function.
- Social Engagement and Community: Cycling can be done alone or as part of a group, providing opportunities for social engagement and community involvement. Joining cycling groups or clubs can offer support, encouragement, and the chance to connect with other people.
- Weight Management: Regular cycling can contribute to weight management and help you maintain a healthy

body weight. Excess weight can also put alot strain on the joints and muscles, exacerbating fibromyalgia symptoms. Cycling can help promote a healthy body composition, which may help alleviate pain and improve your overall quality of life.

When it comes to cycling, like any exercise program, you should begin slowly and gradually increase the intensity and duration of your sessions based on your ability. Remember to always listen to your body and make adjustments as needed.

Dancing

Adding some dance moves to your routine can be enjoyable and beneficial. Research suggests that dancing might improve how you process pain and is a fun social activity. Here's how dancing can help you:

- Low-Impact Exercise: Dancing can be adapted to different intensity levels and styles, making it a flexible and low-impact exercise option. It lets you choose movements that are comfortable for your body and minimizes stress on your joints and muscles.
- Cardiovascular Health: Dancing is a form of aerobic exercise that can improve your cardiovascular health by increasing your heart rate. Regular dance sessions are known to enhance your lung capacity, boost blood circulation, and improve your cardiovascular endurance. This, in turn, can help combat feelings of fatigue and increase your energy levels. So, if you want

to stay fit and healthy, dancing is a great physical activity that you should try.

- Muscle Strength and Endurance: Dancing involves various rhythmic movements that engage multiple muscle groups throughout your body. It helps strengthen and tone your muscles, including the legs, core, and upper body. Building strength and endurance through dancing can also help alleviate muscle weakness.
- Flexibility and Range of Motion: Dancing incorporates a wide range of movements that can improve your flexibility and increase joint mobility. Regular dance practices can help enhance the range of motion in your joints, reduce stiffness, and improve overall mobility. This can be particularly beneficial if you often struggle with joint pain and limited flexibility.
- Balance and Coordination: Dancing requires coordination, balance, and body awareness. Practicing various dance moves can improve your coordination skills, enhance balance, and develop a better sense of body control. It can help reduce your risk of falling and improve overall stability, especially if you experience balance issues.
- Stress Relief and Mood Enhancement: Dancing can be a fun and uplifting activity that promotes stress relief and improves your mood. The release of endorphins during dancing can help reduce feelings of stress, depression, and anxiety while providing you with a creative outlet and offering a sense of joy and self-expression.

- Social Engagement and Community: Participating in dance classes or joining dance groups can provide social engagement and a sense of community. Dancing with others who share similar interests can create a supportive environment, foster connections, and offer opportunities for social interaction and friendship.

It's important to choose dance styles and movements that are suitable for your comfort level and physical abilities. Start gradually and listen to your body, making modifications as necessary.

Stretching Exercises

Stretching can increase flexibility, reduce tension, and improve range of motion. Incorporate gentle stretching exercises for major muscle groups, focusing on areas that commonly experience tightness or discomfort.

Here's an example of a simple neck stretch that can help you:

- Sit or stand in a comfortable position with your back straight.
- Tilt your head gently to one side, bringing your ear towards your shoulder.
- Hold the stretch for 15-30 seconds, feeling a gentle stretch along the opposite side of your neck.
- Return your head to the center and repeat the stretch on the other side.
- Repeat the stretch 2-3 times on each side.

This neck stretch can help relieve tension and stiffness in your neck and shoulders, which are common areas of discomfort for fibromyalgia warriors. It's important to remember to perform stretches slowly and gently without bouncing or forcing movement. Remember that you can adjust or discontinue the stretch if you experience any pain or discomfort.

Strength Training

Research shows that low-, moderate, or high-intensity strength training could be safe if you live with fibromyalgia. In fact, a recent study discovered that women with fibromyalgia actually prefer training with heavier loads and fewer repetitions (Andersson et al., 2021). But, as with any exercise regimen, it is a good idea to consult your healthcare provider first. Once you get the green light, you can consider starting a gradual strength-training program.

For fibromyalgia warriors, strength-training exercises can also be incredibly beneficial. Building strength might not only increase muscle power but also helps reduce fibromyalgia pain and lessen fatigue.

Strength exercises help build muscle strength and improve overall physical function. You can choose to work with light weights, resistance bands, or bodyweight exercises to target different muscle groups. Remember to start with low resistance and gradually progress as tolerated.

Mind-body exercises

Mind-body practices, which blend movement, meditation, and controlled breathing. A couple of gentle methods include:

- Yoga: Studies have highlighted yoga's potential in aiding those with fibromyalgia. In a small-scale study, women with the conditional practiced daily yoga for six weeks and reported improved pain, fatigue, sleep quality, mood, and self-confidence (Andersson et al., 2021). However, evidence of yoga's effectiveness remains varied.
- Tai chi: Similar to yoga, tai chi shows promise in easing both physical and mental symptoms associated with fibromyalgia. Recent research suggests that tai chi is as effective as aerobics, potentially leading to an enhanced quality of life (Andersson et al., 2021). Nonetheless, more comprehensive studies are needed to solidify these findings.

EXERCISING WITH FIBROMYALGIA: HOW TO GET STARTED

There are most certainly different strokes for different folks when it comes to fibromyalgia. When it comes to living with fibromyalgia, it is important to find exercises that work for you. What worked well for another fibromyalgia warrior might not work for you. Do not give up hope; keep pushing forward until you find an exercise routine that works for you. Before embarking on any exercise routine, it may be a good idea for you to have a chat with your healthcare provider to get the green light.

Here are a few tips to consider along your fitness adventure:

- Start gently. Some people find that their fibromyalgia symptoms can act up with exercise, particularly when trying new activities. Begin slowly with low-impact exercises and gradually increase the intensity over time.
- Keep an eye on how your body reacts to different exercises. Pay attention to how you feel while you are trying different activities. By observing your body's responses, you can pick the best, hopefully pain-free, workouts for you.
- Adjust your workouts as needed. Many exercises, such as tai chi and yoga, offer modifications, allowing you to tailor moves based on your abilities and comfort.
- Remember, some movement is better than none. You might not always squeeze in a full workout, but every bit of movement counts. A short walk or daily activities like gardening or shopping also count as physical activity.
- Strive for consistency. Making physical activity, even small efforts, part of your daily routine is key to seeing better results.
- Listen to your body and rest when needed. Always give yourself time to recover after exercising.
- Be gentle with yourself. Discovering the right fitness routine is a process of trial and error, especially when dealing with chronic pain and other fibromyalgia

symptoms. Be compassionate and kind to yourself along this journey.

While dealing with fibromyalgia, exercising can indeed be a challenge due to the chronic pain it brings. Yet, staying active might be the key to managing those symptoms. Research points to the benefits of aerobics and strength training (Mayo Clinic Staff, 2018). However, there is no single perfect exercise routine for fibromyalgia.

TIPS FOR MOVING WITH FIBROMYALGIA

Fibromyalgia can make it challenging to move around and perform daily activities. However, with the help of some careful planning and thoughtful strategies, it is possible to make moving with fibromyalgia more manageable. By taking steps to reduce pain and fatigue, pacing yourself, and engaging in gentle exercise, you can enjoy a better, active, and fulfilling lifestyle despite the challenges posed by fibromyalgia.

Here are a few strategies to consider:

- Accept some discomfort: Acknowledging and accepting a certain degree of pain is okay. Understanding your body's signals is crucial for maintaining a sustainable routine.
- Avoid overexertion: Steer clear of overdoing it. Pay attention to your body and avoid activities that lead to excessive strain.

- Embrace your limits: It is important to acknowledge and respect your body's limits. Listen to what your body tells you and work within those boundaries.
- Explore new activities: Consider low-impact exercises or activities that are gentler on your body. Water aerobics, tai chi, or gentle yoga might be great options to explore.
- Find balance: Sometimes, compromise is key. It is okay to adjust your routine or activities to accommodate your body's needs.
- Medication adherence: Do not skip or avoid your prescribed medications. They are important in managing symptoms and enabling a more active lifestyle.
- Persistence pays off: Do not give up. Keep exploring and finding what works best for you. It might take time, but persistence can lead to discovering the right balance.
- Prioritize energy: Save your energy for things that truly matter to you. Choose activities that bring you joy and peace and conserve your energy for those moments.
- Right footwear matters: Invest in comfortable, supportive footwear. Good shoes can significantly reduce strain on your body.
- Take it easy: Dial down the intensity, pace yourself, and avoid pushing too hard. Small but consistent efforts can make a huge difference without exacerbating symptoms.

Living with fibromyalgia can be a challenging and unique journey for each person affected by it. As such, it is important to seek guidance and advice from your healthcare provider, who can provide personalized strategies and recommendations tailored to your specific needs. Remember to prioritize your own well-being and be kind to yourself throughout this process. It can be difficult, but take things one step at a time and remember that you are doing great. With the right support and self-care, it is possible to manage fibromyalgia and live a fulfilling life.

In this chapter, *Movement as Medicine*, you looked into the incredible benefits of physical activity beyond just fitness. It emphasizes how movement is vital for our physical health and deeply intertwined with our mental and emotional well-being. It highlights how engaging in various forms of movement, whether through exercise, dance or even simply taking a stroll, positively impacts our overall health.

The chapter stresses the concept that movement is indeed a form of medicine, improving mood, reducing stress, and enhancing cognitive function. It supports the idea that integrating movement into our daily routines is pivotal for a holistic approach to well-being.

The next chapter, *Your Sanctuary*, is a natural extension of the discourse on well-being. This chapter dives into the significance of creating spaces and practices that foster inner peace and mental tranquility. It delves into how our physical and mental environment contributes to our overall wellness.

Your Sanctuary looks into how nurturing spaces, whether at home or in your mind, can act as havens for relaxation, rejuvenation, and emotional balance. It explores the significance of creating environments that promote mental peace and harmony, ultimately contributing to a healthier, more balanced life.

Exploring the impact of surroundings and mental spaces on well-being, Your Sanctuary continues the conversation on holistic health sparked by Movement as Medicine. This chapter delves into how creating personal sanctuaries can significantly contribute to your mental health, providing insights and practical steps to establish a tranquil haven in your life.

The transition from *Movement as Medicine* to *Your Sanctuary* allows you to seamlessly continue your journey toward comprehensive well-being, expanding your understanding of how movement and mindful spaces are interconnected in nurturing a healthier and more balanced life.

Share Your Story, Share Your Strength

"The greatest gift you can give someone is your own personal development."

— JIM ROHN

Hey there! You know, they say the greatest joy in life comes from helping others. And guess what? It's true! When we share our experiences, we can make a huge difference in someone else's life, especially when it comes to something as challenging as fibromyalgia.

I've got a little favour to ask you... Would you be willing to help someone you might never meet? Imagine a person just like you, facing the struggles of fibromyalgia, searching for answers and hope. That's who you can help today!

Our goal with "Fibromyalgia Unraveled" is to reach out to as many people as possible who are navigating through this condition. We want to offer them knowledge, hope, and a sense of community. And the only way we can do this is with your help.

You see, when you leave a review for this book, you're not just writing a few sentences. You're giving a voice to your own journey with fibromyalgia. Your words can guide, inspire, and comfort someone else who's in the thick of their battle. By sharing your thoughts, you become a beacon of hope for another Fibro Warrior.

Here's what you can do: take a moment (just a minute or two) to leave a review. It doesn't cost a thing, but the value it brings could be life-changing for someone else. Your review could be the reason someone feels less alone, gets the push to try a new strategy, or finds the strength to keep fighting.

Ready to make a difference? It's super easy! Just scan the QR code below to leave your review:

By helping out, you're not just a reader; you become part of our fibromyalgia community. Together, we can make each day a little brighter, a little easier for those facing this challenge.

I can't wait to continue this journey with you. There are so many more insights and strategies to share in the upcoming chapters. And remember, each step you take in managing fibromyalgia not only helps you but also lights the way for others.

Thank you so much for your kindness and generosity. Let's keep making a positive impact, one word at a time.

Your friend and fellow Fibro Warrior, Courtney Dale

P.S. Remember, sharing knowledge is like sharing light – it brightens everyone's path. If you think this book could help another Fibro Warrior, don't hesitate to pass it along. Let's spread hope and healing together!

6

YOUR SANCTUARY

> Our inner space and our peace of mind are affected by our outer space.
>
> — THICH NHAT HANH

THE PSYCHOLOGY OF SPACE

Your life is intricately woven into the tapestry of the spaces that you inhabit. From the corners of your home to your workplace cubicles and the wide expanse of public places, different environments are more than physical spaces - they are vibrant contributors to your mental and emotional well-being.

Carl Jung once profoundly remarked, "Your vision will become clear only when you can look into your heart. Who looks outside, dreams; who looks inside, awakes." This sentiment poignantly reflects the profound interconnectedness between your external environment and internal state.

Your surroundings have an incredible impact on your psychological well-being. Take your home, for instance - it is not just a building but an extension of your inner self. Your home's arrangement, color scheme, and decor can significantly influence your emotions, thoughts, and behaviors. A cluttered or disorganized space often leads to a cluttered and anxious mind. Conversely, a tidy, aesthetically pleasing environment can nurture a sense of calm and clarity within you.

Likewise, your workplace plays a pivotal role in your mental health. The design, layout, and atmosphere of your work environment affect your stress levels, productivity, and overall job satisfaction. A noisy or chaotic workplace can elevate stress and disrupt focus, while a well-organized and tranquil space can foster concentration and creativity.

Public spaces, too, bear immense significance in your psychological well-being. They are physical locations and landscapes that evoke emotions and trigger memories. For example, the aroma of a certain food or the sight of a familiar landmark might instantly transport us back to cherished memories. Natural settings like parks and gardens also have a remarkable ability to reduce your stress and elevate your mood.

The psychology behind how your surroundings affect you is multifaceted. Your senses-sight, smell, sound, touch, and taste-are intimately linked to your emotions and memories. A particular smell or piece of music can evoke powerful emotions or nostalgic memories. This deep connection explains why aromatherapy can have calming effects and why specific sounds can soothe or disturb you.

Moreover, the impact of your environment on your sleep patterns is undeniable. Factors like ambient noise, temperature, and light significantly influence the quality of your sleep. A quiet, dark, and comfortably cool environment is conducive to restful sleep. Disruptions like street noise, bright lights, or uncomfortable temperatures can lead to sleep disturbances and affect overall well-being.

Understanding this intricate connection between your surroundings and your mental and emotional state empowers you to make informed choices about your environment. You can positively impact your emotional and mental health by deliberately curating spaces that promote tranquility, comfort, and positivity.

In the context of stress, an environment that nurtures calmness and order can act as a buffer against daily life stressors. A clutter-free, organized space can create a sense of control and reduce overwhelming feelings. The right ambiance can offer a sanctuary amidst chaos, allowing for moments of solace and rejuvenation.

Similarly, a well-designed workplace that fosters collaboration, provides visual interest, and allows personalization can improve job satisfaction and overall well-being. Public spaces designed with an emphasis on comfort, safety, and natural elements can also create a sense of community and enhance the experience for all who frequent them.

In essence, your external environment significantly influences your internal state. Crafting spaces that positively impact mental and emotional well-being requires recognition of the bond between the two. By creating environments that resonate with your senses, evoke positive emotions, and encourage tranquility, you can harness the power of your surroundings to lead more fulfilling and balanced lives.

FIBROMYALGIA AND SENSITIVITIES

For people living with fibromyalgia, the daily experience extends far beyond the visible symptoms. Often, heightened sensitivities play a significant role in your lives, impacting your interaction with the environment. Sensitivity to various stimuli like noise, light, and temperature is a common facet of fibromyalgia and, in turn, makes the environment a crucial factor in this invisible illness.

The heightened sensitivities experienced by people with fibromyalgia can be overwhelming and challenging to navigate. Sensitivity to noise, for instance, can be particularly distressing. Loud or sudden noises that others might barely notice can trigger discomfort or even pain for someone with fibromyalgia. What might be perceived as background noise to many can, for someone with this condition, feel amplified and stressful.

Similarly, sensitivity to light becomes a pertinent concern. Harsh lighting, bright, flickering lights, or even sudden changes in lighting conditions can result in discomfort, headaches, or migraines for people with fibromyalgia. This sensitivity often dictates the choice of environments and even the timing of outdoor activities, as exposure to specific light conditions, can significantly impact their well-being.

Temperature sensitivity is another challenge. Extreme heat or cold can aggravate the symptoms of fibromyalgia, intensifying pain and discomfort. This sensitivity often requires people to control their immediate environment, including room temperature, clothing choices, and the duration of exposure to different temperatures.

The environment becomes even more crucial for people with fibromyalgia due to these heightened sensitivities. Designing and curating spaces that accommodate these sensitivities becomes a necessity rather than a luxury. For those with fibromyalgia, the right environment can act as a protective shield against triggers, allowing them to manage their symptoms and function more comfortably.

Creating an environment that caters to these sensitivities involves several considerations. Soft, diffused lighting can significantly reduce discomfort and mitigate the risk of triggering migraines or headaches. Controlling the level and type of lighting in a space becomes crucial for those with fibromyalgia.

Soundproofing or the use of soothing background noise can be hugely beneficial in reducing the impact of external noises. This can include using white noise machines, sound-absorbing materials, or creating an environment that minimizes sudden or loud sounds.

Temperature control is vital for those with fibromyalgia. Ensuring the room temperature is comfortable and consistent helps manage discomfort associated with temperature fluctuations. This often involves using heating or cooling systems that allow precise environmental control.

The challenge lies not only in adapting one's own home but also in seeking environments outside the home that can accommodate these sensitivities. Public spaces, workplaces, or social settings may present hurdles due to their often unpredictable or uncontrollable sensory elements.

Understanding these heightened sensitivities and their impact on people with fibromyalgia emphasizes the importance of creating supportive environments. By considering and addressing these sensitivities in the design and maintenance of spaces, whether at home or in public, we can significantly enhance the quality of life for those living with fibromyalgia. Creating supportive environments can act as a catalyst for their comfort, minimizing triggers and contributing to an improved overall sense of well-being.

A Space that Heals

Creating a personal sanctuary within your home is like weaving a nurturing cocoon enveloping you in tranquility, offering solace and rejuvenation. This space, dedicated to relaxation, meditation, or simply 'me time,' becomes your haven—a place where the world's chaos melts away, and peace and comfort take center stage.

Defining the Space

The first step is to choose the right space for your sanctuary. It doesn't have to be vast or extravagant. It could be a cozy corner by a window, a peaceful nook in your bedroom, or a small area in the living room. Find a spot that speaks to your soul, where you can unwind and feel at ease.

Declutter and Simplify Your Life

Decluttering is the magical act of freeing both your space and your mind. Simplify by discerning what truly brings you joy and peace. Keep only the essentials and those items that resonate with your heart. A clutter-free space cultivates a clutter-free mind, making room for tranquility.

Choose the Right Colors

Colors wield incredible power over our emotions. Opt for calming tones that resonate with you—soft blues, serene greens, or warm, earthy hues. Experiment with combinations until you find a palette that speaks to your inner sense of peace.

Decorate with Meaning

Infuse your sanctuary with items that hold significance or reflect your passions. It could be a piece of art that moves you, a cherished family heirloom, or something collected from your travels. These meaningful touches breathe life into your space and infuse it with warmth.

Invite Nature In

Bringing elements of nature indoors adds a soothing touch to your sanctuary. Consider houseplants that not only freshen the air but also lend a sense of serenity. Even small succulents or potted herbs can enliven the space. Natural elements connect us to the peaceful outdoors, fostering a serene environment.

Use Sounds that Soothe

The right sounds can create an ambiance of peace. Explore soothing nature sounds or calming music to infuse your sanctuary with tranquility. Consider using apps or playlists designed for relaxation or meditation to create an atmosphere that eases your mind.

Set the Mood with Lighting

Lighting is a cornerstone in establishing the atmosphere of your sanctuary. Soft, gentle, and warm lighting can create a cozy ambiance. Lamps with delicate hues or candles can cast a serene glow. Embrace natural light during the day to illuminate your space with warmth.

Support the Senses

Textures and aromas are often underestimated yet critical elements of a soothing sanctuary. Soft textures like plush pillows, cozy blankets, or a soft rug can invite comfort. Aromatherapy through candles, essential oil diffusers, or incense can infuse the air with scents that calm and uplift your spirits.

Remember, your personal sanctuary is a canvas for your well-being. Experiment, adjust, and mold it to suit your preferences and needs. Your space should be as unique as you are and evolve as you do. The journey of creating your sanctuary is an exploration of self-care and an invitation to indulge in moments of relaxation and rejuvenation.

Maintain your space with care and love. Keep it fresh with items that inspire you and bring you joy. Cherish the moments you spend within it, as these moments are gifts to your well-being and your soul. Embrace this haven within your home—a place where you can unwind, recharge, and find peace amidst life's journey.

NATURE'S THERAPY

Nature, with its boundless beauty and serenity, holds remarkable healing powers, especially for those navigating the tumultuous path of chronic pain. The therapeutic effects of nature are profound, offering solace, comfort, and a rejuvenating embrace that can be particularly transformative for people experiencing persistent pain.

For those grappling with chronic pain, nature serves as a tranquil haven, providing relief and respite from the trials of everyday life. Immersing oneself in natural environments, whether a serene forest, a calming beach, or a vibrant garden, can be a powerful form of therapy. The sights, sounds, and scents of nature have an innate ability to soothe both the body and the mind.

The natural world has a mesmerizing way of engaging our senses. The lush greenery, vibrant colors, and gentle movements of leaves in the wind are visually captivating. These visual stimuli not only offer a picturesque setting but also divert attention away from pain, fostering a sense of calm and distraction.

The sounds of nature—a bubbling brook, birdsong, rustling leaves—create a symphony that acts as a balm for the soul. These gentle, harmonious sounds are soothing and alleviate stress and anxiety. They draw attention away from the body's discomfort, offering a space for the mind to wander and find solace.

Furthermore, the scents of nature, from the earthy aroma of the forest to the salty air by the ocean, have an uncanny ability to calm and rejuvenate. These natural fragrances stimulate the olfactory senses, promoting relaxation and an overall sense of well-being.

The therapeutic effects of nature for chronic pain extend beyond mere distraction or relaxation. Studies have shown that spending time in natural environments can reduce pain perception (Pattemore, 2022). The calming effects of nature can lower stress, subsequently decreasing the intensity of pain experienced by individuals.

Moreover, nature serves as a canvas for physical activity and gentle exercise, which can be beneficial for managing chronic pain. Activities like walking, gentle yoga, or simply being outside and moving at one's own pace can aid in increasing mobility and reducing discomfort associated with chronic pain.

There is also evidence suggesting that exposure to natural light and fresh air has positive effects on one's mood and sleep patterns. Improved mood and better sleep are crucial components in managing chronic pain, as they can positively impact an individual's overall well-being.

The connection with nature offers a holistic approach to healing. It provides an opportunity to step away from the confinement of four walls and embrace the vastness of the outdoors. This connection with the natural world not only offers physical relief but also fosters a sense of emotional and spiritual well-being.

It's crucial to acknowledge that the therapeutic effects of nature for chronic pain are not a one-size-fits-all solution. However, for many people, integrating nature into their lives, whether through regular walks in the park, spending time in their garden, or planning nature-based outings, can provide a significant sense of relief and comfort.

Nature's therapy is a gift available to us all. Embracing the outdoors, immersing ourselves in its wonders, and finding solace in its beauty can be a cornerstone in managing chronic pain, providing a sanctuary of peace and healing amidst life's challenges.

VISIT URBAN SPACES.

For city dwellers, navigating the bustling urban landscape means being enveloped in a whirlwind of activity and concrete. Amidst the hustle and bustle, urban green spaces, such as parks, community gardens, and even green rooftops, emerge as crucial sanctuaries, offering a breath of fresh air and a momentary escape from the stressors of city life.

Parks, the emerald gems nestled within urban jungles, are vital havens for those seeking refuge from the constant motion of the city. These green spaces provide a reprieve from the concrete jungle, allowing people to unwind, recharge, and reconnect with nature within the city limits. Parks offer various activities, from peaceful strolls and picnics to recreational sports, catering to the varied needs of city dwellers seeking relaxation and rejuvenation.

Community gardens, with their vibrant patches of greenery amidst urban blocks, play an essential role in fostering a sense of community and serenity. These spaces not only offer the therapeutic benefits of nurturing plants but also provide a communal hub for interaction and shared gardening experiences. The act of gardening in itself has been shown to reduce stress and promote a sense of well-being, making community gardens vital oases in the urban landscape.

Even green rooftops, whether atop skyscrapers or smaller buildings, contribute to the urban landscape's respite. These elevated green spaces offer a unique opportunity for relaxation and connection with nature during the urban hustle. They provide a tranquil setting for city dwellers to enjoy nature's beauty, offering a panoramic view of greenery against the backdrop of the cityscape.

The benefits of these urban green spaces are manifold. Beyond their aesthetic appeal, they play a crucial role in enhancing the well-being of city residents. Having access to green spaces has been linked to better overall mental health, lower stress levels, and increased happiness. Time spent in these areas offers a reprieve from the concrete monotony, allowing people to recharge and reconnect with nature, even in the heart of a bustling city.

Research suggests that spending time outside in green spaces within urban settings can lower stress hormones, reduce symptoms of anxiety and depression, and improve overall mental well-being (Chen et al., 2021). These green pockets provide a much-needed connection to nature, fostering a sense of calm and tranquility amidst the urban chaos.

Furthermore, these green spaces offer opportunities for physical activities, such as walking, jogging, or yoga, contributing to improved physical health and fitness. Being in these natural environments encourages people to engage in outdoor activities that may not be as easily accessible within the confines of the city.

The significance of urban green spaces cannot be overstated. They act as vital sanctuaries within the urban environment, providing a natural haven that rejuvenates and uplifts. As cities continue to grow and urban life becomes increasingly fast-paced, the presence and accessibility of these green spaces become indispensable for the well-being and quality of life of city residents.

By promoting the creation and maintenance of these urban oases, city planners and communities can foster a harmonious balance between urban development and the preservation of natural environments, ensuring that city residents have access to the restorative power of nature amidst the concrete landscape.

Care for Pets at Home.

Pets, with their boundless affection and unwavering loyalty, have an incredible knack for soothing not only the soul but also the body. In the context of conditions like fibromyalgia, where pain management and emotional well-being are paramount, the presence of pets offers a unique form of therapy that goes beyond words.

The emotional bond between people with fibromyalgia and their pets is a treasure trove of comfort and understanding. Animals have an innate ability to sense their owner's emotional state, offering companionship and solace during difficult times. Their constant companionship creates a profound sense of support, providing an emotional anchor that can be profoundly reassuring, particularly on days when coping with chronic pain seems impossible.

The therapeutic effects of pets are far-reaching. The mere act of petting an animal, whether it's a gentle stroke of fur or a cuddle, releases endorphins—the body's natural pain relievers. This release of feel-good hormones can aid in managing pain and reducing discomfort associated with fibromyalgia. The presence of a beloved pet can alleviate stress, reducing the perception of pain and promoting relaxation.

Moreover, the bond formed with pets can significantly reduce feelings of isolation and loneliness often experienced by people dealing with chronic pain conditions. Pets offer unconditional love and an unwavering presence, fostering a sense of connection and companionship. Their playful antics and loving nature serve as a source of joy and distraction from the trials of managing pain.

The physical benefits of having a pet are equally significant. Daily interactions with pets often encourage physical activity. Walking your dog, playing with a cat, or engaging in pet care routines can promote movement and exercise, which is crucial for managing pain and maintaining mobility. This physical activity, even in small doses, can contribute to better overall physical health and fitness.

Moreover, the routine and responsibility of caring for your pet can offer a sense of purpose and structure to an individual's day, adding a valuable sense of normalcy to life despite the challenges posed by chronic pain.

The emotional support pets provide goes hand in hand with the bond formed, nurturing a positive state of mind. This emotional balance can be vital in managing the emotional toll that comes with chronic pain conditions like fibromyalgia. The stress reduction and emotional support offered by pets can positively impact mental health, offering a sense of peace and well-being amidst the challenges of pain management.

Overall, the presence of pets in the lives of people managing fibromyalgia offers a multifaceted form of therapy. Their unwavering companionship, emotional support, and the physical benefits derived from interactions foster a sense of comfort and joy. For those navigating the complex journey of pain management, pets play an integral role, offering a unique and invaluable source of solace, understanding, and unwavering love.

EMBRACING THE HEALING EMBRACE OF NATURE: FOREST BATHING AND GROUNDING FOR YOUR WELL-BEING

Nature, with its calming embrace and boundless tranquility, has a remarkable ability to heal both the body and the soul. Practices like forest bathing and grounding are nature-based therapies that offer a profound connection to the Earth, enhancing well-being and offering a sanctuary away from the rush of daily life.

What is Forest Bathing?

Forest bathing, or Shinrin-yoku, is a Japanese practice that involves immersing oneself in a forest environment. It's not about hiking or exercise but about slowing down and engaging the senses in nature. The practice invites people to mindfully absorb the natural atmosphere, taking in the sights, sounds, and scents of the forest, allowing nature to work its magic on the mind and body.

Benefits of Forest Bathing

Studies have shown the transformative effects of forest therapy (Weir, 2020). Participants reported significant decreases in pain and depression, alongside increased quality of life. Forest therapy acts as an effective intervention, relieving both psychological and physiological pain. The forest environment has been linked to reduced stress, improved mood, and better overall well-being.

How to Practice Forest Bathing

To engage in forest bathing:

1. Find a quiet forest or natural area.
2. Slow down, be present, and engage your senses.
3. Take a slow and mindful walk, paying attention to the sounds of singing birds, rustling leaves, and fragrant forest scents.
4. Take your time, breathe deeply, and allow the calming aura of nature to envelop you.

What is Grounding/Earthing?

Grounding, or earthing, involves direct physical contact with the Earth's surface. This practice reconnects people with the Earth's electrons by walking barefoot, lying on the ground, or sitting directly on the Earth. The Earth's surface provides an abundant supply of free electrons, which can positively influence our physiological processes.

Benefits of Grounding

Direct contact with the Earth's surface can influence physiological processes, potentially reducing pain and inflammation, improving sleep, and enhancing overall well-being. Research suggests that grounding can help balance the body's electrical charge, counteracting the effects of positive electrons accumulated from modern lifestyles, such as wearing shoes and living in insulated homes (*What Is Earthing Grounding & Can It Transform Your Health?* 2015).

How to Ground Yourself

Grounding is simple. Spend time barefoot on natural surfaces like grass, sand, or soil. Walk barefoot in the park, stand on the beach, or sit on the ground. Allow your skin to connect directly with the Earth, absorbing its natural energy.

Embracing these practices is an invitation to engage with nature's healing power. Forest bathing and grounding offer you the opportunity to disconnect from the chaos of everyday life and reconnect with the serene energy of the Earth. It is a chance to slow down, breathe deeply, and allow nature to embrace you, offering solace and rejuvenation in its natural embrace.

In the chapter *Your Sanctuary*, the focal point revolves around creating a personal haven within the home. The essence of this chapter is centered on the idea of curating a space dedicated to relaxation, meditation, and emotional rejuvenation. It emphasizes the importance of defining a space, decluttering, choosing suitable colors, decorating with meaning, inviting nature in, and supporting the senses with soothing elements like sounds, lighting, textures, and aromas.

The main premise is that by intentionally crafting a space within your home to align with your well-being, you can create a sanctuary that fosters tranquility and reduces stress. This haven acts as a retreat from the demands of everyday life, offering a cocoon of peace and comfort tailored to your preferences.

Moving forward, the upcoming chapter, *Sounds That Heal,* is a logical continuation of the theme of nurturing well-being within one's personal space. It delves into the profound influence of sounds on our mental and emotional states. It explores how certain sounds can have therapeutic effects, soothing the mind and body.

The chapter expands upon how specific auditory elements, from gentle music to nature sounds, can foster relaxation, alleviate stress, and contribute to overall wellness. It highlights the significance of sound in creating an atmosphere conducive to healing and tranquility within our living spaces. The focus on sounds that heal continues the journey of crafting an environment dedicated to enhancing our well-being, offering a deeper understanding of how auditory elements contribute to our sanctuary and furthering our exploration of creating spaces that soothe the soul.

Your Sanctuary is more than just a space; it's an oasis within your home designed specifically for relaxation, meditation, and personal rejuvenation. This chapter is about curating a haven that speaks directly to your soul, fostering tranquility and calmness amidst the chaos of daily life.

The concept of *Your Sanctuary* revolves around the deliberate creation of a space dedicated to your well-being. It begins with defining a space within your home, whether a cozy nook, a peaceful corner by a window, or a special area in your living room. The goal is to carve out a place that feels uniquely yours, allowing for moments of solace and comfort.

Decluttering and simplifying your space is a cornerstone of this sanctuary. Clearing out unnecessary items and surrounding yourself with things that bring you joy creates a sense of calm and clarity. Choosing the right colors that resonate with your soul is also key. Soft blues, serene greens, or warm, earthy hues can help set a peaceful ambiance.

Decorating with meaning adds depth and warmth to your sanctuary. It's about infusing the space with items that hold significance or reflect your passions. Meaningful decor elements evoke positive emotions and create an inviting environment.

Inviting nature into your sanctuary is a game-changer. Whether through houseplants, natural materials, or glimpses of the outdoors, nature brings a calming and soothing touch, connecting you to the serenity of the natural world.

Supporting the senses through sounds that soothe is equally crucial. Creating an atmosphere with gentle music, nature sounds, or white noise can work wonders in promoting relaxation and reducing stress. Lighting is another powerful tool in setting the mood. Soft, warm lighting creates a cozy ambiance, allowing for moments of calmness and serenity.

But it's not just about sight and sound. Textures and aromas play a significant role in your sanctuary. Soft, cozy textures like plush pillows and comforting blankets create an inviting space. Aromatherapy through candles or essential oils can infuse the air with scents that calm and uplift your spirits.

Your sanctuary is a space of self-care, a retreat where you can leave the world's stresses at the door and simply be. It's a canvas for your well-being, ever-evolving as you do. The journey of creating "Your Sanctuary" is a personal exploration of what brings you comfort, peace, and joy, offering a haven that resonates with your soul.

By embracing the idea of your sanctuary, you invite moments of respite, allowing yourself to breathe and reconnect amidst life's hustle. Your sanctuary is not just a physical space; it's a mindset—a commitment to your well-being. Your sanctuary is a constant reminder that amidst the chaos, there's always a place of peace waiting for you within your own home.

7

SOUNDS THAT HEAL

66 Music can heal the wounds which medicine cannot touch."

— DEBASISH MRIDHA

W elcome to a harmonious journey into the world of music and its remarkable potential in managing fibromyalgia symptoms. In this chapter, you will explore music's transformative and therapeutic effects, delving into the science behind music therapy and how it can offer solace and relief for those navigating the challenges of fibromyalgia.

The healing power of music is far-reaching and often underestimated. As you navigate the complexities of fibromyalgia, discovering how music can be harnessed as a tool for comfort and support is an enlightening adventure. You will uncover the profound impact of melodies and rhythms on your physical and emotional well-being, unraveling the science behind how music therapy can significantly alleviate symptoms and contribute to overall wellness.

Moreover, this chapter offers you a guide to craft your personalized healing playlists. By understanding the therapeutic effects of different musical elements, we aim to assist in curating a selection of songs and sounds that resonate with people's experiences and aid in managing fibromyalgia symptoms. This personalized approach empowers you to tailor your musical journey toward alleviating discomfort, reducing stress, and fostering moments of respite.

As you continue to embark on this musical voyage, we invite you to uncover the potential of music therapy, exploring how melodies and rhythms can be harnessed to support your well-being, uplift your spirits, and offer a gentle embrace during fibromyalgia trials. So, let the symphony of healing begin as we unravel the therapeutic influence of music in managing fibromyalgia symptoms, ultimately aiming to harmonize your path toward a more comfortable and balanced life.

THE POWER OF SOUND AND MUSIC

Music and sound, often perceived as music to your ears, hold profound therapeutic potential beyond simple enjoyment. By delving into the intersection of sound and human health, you will uncover the intricate science behind sound therapy and music's incredible impact on your well-being.

The Science Behind Sound Therapy

Sound therapy, a practice rooted in ancient healing traditions, involves using various sound frequencies to restore balance and promote healing in the body. It operates on the understanding that specific sound vibrations can influence your physical, emotional, and mental well-being. The fundamentals of sound and its effects on the human body lie in the concept of resonance, where sound vibrations interact with the body's vibrational patterns to induce a state of relaxation and harmony.

The science behind sound healing emphasizes the mechanisms through which sound vibrations impact the body. Sound healing operates on the principle that different frequencies. It can stimulate the release of endorphins, supporting pain relief and reducing stress, thereby promoting overall well-being. Encompassing practices like binaural beats, singing bowls, or sound baths, sound therapy aims to restore equilibrium within the body and mind through the harmonious interaction of sound waves.

The Impact of Music on Our Psyche and Physiology

Music, a universal language, has a profound impact on the human psyche and physiology. Listening to music you love triggers the release of neurotransmitters like dopamine, fostering a sense of pleasure and joy. This dopamine release is pivotal in alleviating pain, reducing stress, and elevating mood.

The neurophysiological responses to music are diverse and fascinating. Entrainment effects, wherein your brain waves synchronize with the rhythm of music, can induce a state of calm and relaxation. Music also regulates emotional responses, impacting heart rate, blood pressure, and respiration, fostering a sense of balance and tranquility.

Variations in musical elements such as tempo, rhythm, and melody are pivotal in influencing the body and mind. Temponce: the tempo can invigorate or soothe, while rhythm impacts your physical movements and emotional state. Melody and harmonies evoke emotions, further contributing to the regulation of mood.

The influence of music extends to reducing stress and anxiety. Listening to calming melodies can significantly lower cortisol levels, the hormone associated with stress, thus providing a calming effect.

Additionally, music serves as a powerful tool for pain management, reducing the perception of pain and promoting comfort.

Music As A Holistic Approach To Managing Symptoms, Especially Relevant For Fibromyalgia Patients

The potential of music as a non-invasive, holistic approach to managing symptoms, particularly for people navigating conditions like fibromyalgia, is truly remarkable. The multifaceted impact of music therapy, ranging from emotional regulation to pain management, offers a holistic approach to enhance overall well-being.

For fibromyalgia patients, music emerges as a beacon of hope amidst the challenges of chronic pain. By embracing music therapy, you can explore a non-pharmacological method that not only aids in managing pain but also offers emotional solace and stress reduction. This holistic approach resonates with the holistic management philosophy of fibromyalgia, providing people with an additional tool for enhancing their quality of life.

The transformative influence of sound and music on your well-being is both powerful and accessible. Music, as a non-invasive and versatile tool, holds the potential to play a pivotal role in the holistic management of conditions like fibromyalgia. As you navigate wellness symptoms, let us acknowledge the healing potential of sound and music, harnessing their harmony to soothe your soul and enhance your overall well-being.

SOUND PRACTICES TO TRY

Binaural Beats

In the realm of sound practices, binaural beats stand as a remarkable phenomenon, offering a potential gateway to enhanced well-being. Let us embark on an explorative journey into the mechanics, benefits, and practical use of binaural beats, especially relevant for those navigating the complexities of fibromyalgia.

The Mechanics Of Binaural Beats

Binaural beats are an auditory illusion created by presenting two different frequencies separately to each ear, resulting in a perceived third frequency. The brain then perceives a third tone, which is the mathematical difference between the two frequencies. For example, if one ear receives a tone at 200 Hz and the other at 210 Hz, the brain perceives a binaural beat of 10 Hz.

This phenomenon is a fundamental aspect of how binaural beats work, influencing the brain's frequency patterns and inducing a state of synchronization or "entrainment." Depending on the frequency presented, the brain responds by aligning its brainwave frequencies to the perceived binaural beat, thus promoting relaxation or stimulation.

Benefits of Binaural Beats for Fibromyalgia Patients

For people managing fibromyalgia, the potential benefits of binaural beats are diverse and promising. Better sleep quality is a key advantage, as the synchronization of brainwaves induced by binaural beats can help regulate sleep patterns and induce a state of relaxation, potentially improving sleep quality.

Another significant advantage is reducing stress levels. Binaural beats' calming effect on brainwave activity can potentially lower stress and anxiety, fostering a sense of tranquility and peace.

Entraining brainwave frequencies with binaural beats can also boost energy levels. By aligning brainwave patterns to specific frequencies, individuals might experience increased alertness and focus, promoting an uplift in energy.

Another notable benefit is enhancing mood and well-being. Binaural beats can induce relaxation, potentially triggering the release of endorphins, which contributes to a more positive mood and a sense of well-being.

Pain management is a key aspect relevant to fibromyalgia patients. While research in this area is ongoing, there is potential for binaural beats to contribute to pain reduction. By promoting relaxation and potentially influencing the perception of pain, binaural beats offer a non-invasive approach to managing fibromyalgia symptoms.

Effective Use of Binaural Beats

To effectively utilize binaural beats, listening with stereo headphones is crucial to ensure each ear receives a distinct frequency. Experimenting with different frequencies, typically ranging between 1 to 30 Hz, can help individuals find the beat frequency that works best for their intended outcome, whether it's relaxation, focus, or sleep enhancement.

Engaging in binaural beats in a comfortable, relaxed environment can maximize their potential benefits. Incorporating these beats into a daily routine, especially during times when stress or pain levels are high, may offer a complementary tool for managing fibromyalgia symptoms.

The potential of binaural beats in enhancing well-being, especially for fibromyalgia patients, is both promising and fascinating. Through their ability to influence brainwave patterns and induce a state of relaxation or stimulation, binaural beats offer a unique and non-invasive method to ease symptoms and enhance overall quality of life.

As we embrace the symphony of sound practices, binaural beats stand as a versatile and accessible tool, offering a harmonious pathway to well-being for those seeking relief from the challenges of fibromyalgia.

SOUND BATHS

Immersing into a Sound Bath Session

Picture this: You're nestled in a serene space, enveloped by dimly lit ambiance, the air vibrating with resonant tones that gently caress your senses. This is the immersive experience of a sound bath session—a therapeutic journey that transcends ordinary relaxation, delving into a realm where sound becomes a healing force.

Historical and Cultural Origins of Sound Baths

The concept of sound baths traces its roots back to ancient civilizations, where sound and vibrations were recognized as powerful healing tools. From indigenous cultures to Eastern philosophies, various societies have embraced sound for restoration and balance. In the modern era, these ancient practices have evolved into therapeutic sessions where sounds, such as crystal singing bowls, gongs, and other instruments, are used to create an immersive, meditative experience.

How Sound Baths Work

During a sound bath, instruments emitting different frequencies and harmonics are played, inducing a meditative state. The vibrations produced by these instruments resonate throughout the body, promoting relaxation and mental stillness. The sound waves interact with your body, guiding it towards a state of harmony and balance.

Benefits for Fibromyalgia Patients

For people managing fibromyalgia, sound baths offer a spectrum of potential benefits. The immersive and deeply relaxing nature of the experience can aid in stress reduction, providing a respite from the daily strain of the condition. By promoting relaxation and reducing stress, sound baths are a valuable tool for managing fibromyalgia symptoms.

Practical Tips for Attending a Sound Bath

Before embarking on a sound bath journey, a few considerations are worth noting. Think about any particular sensitivities or needs you might have and discuss them with the facilitator beforehand to ensure a comfortable experience.

The attire for a sound bath should be comfortable and conducive to relaxation. Loose-fitting clothing that will allow for easy movement and comfort is recommended. Many sound bath sessions are conducted while lying down; choosing clothing that facilitates this is ideal.

Regarding what to bring, most sound bath sessions provide yoga mats, blankets, and sometimes eye masks or cushions. However, feel free to bring your own if it enhances your comfort. It's also advisable to avoid heavy meals before the session to ensure you're not uncomfortable while lying down.

Sound baths typically last around 60 to 90 minutes. The facilitator will guide you through the session, playing various instruments and allowing the sounds and vibrations to wash over you.

During the session, you may experience a range of sensations. Some people feel a sense of deep relaxation, while others might notice emotional release or even heightened sensitivity to the sounds. It is a deeply personal experience, and each person may react differently.

Sound baths offer a holistic journey into relaxation and healing, leveraging the power of sound to soothe the mind and body. For fibromyalgia patients, they present an accessible and non-invasive method to seek relief and reduce stress, promoting an environment conducive to managing symptoms. As you prepare for a sound bath, consider these tips to make the experience more comfortable, allowing yourself to immerse fully in the therapeutic sounds and vibrations for a journey towards serenity and well-being.

SOLFEGGIO FREQUENCIES

Exploring the Healing Potential of Solfeggio Frequencies

Solfeggio frequencies represent a series of tones believed to possess unique healing qualities and spiritual resonance. These frequencies, originating from an ancient musical scale, are purported to offer a path to holistic healing and spiritual elevation. While the scientific evidence supporting these claims might be limited, the philosophy behind Solfeggio frequencies revolves around their impact on the body's energy, vibration, and emotional well-being, making them an intriguing subject for exploration.

Understanding the Science Behind Solfeggio Frequencies

Solfeggio frequencies are rooted in the ancient hymn "Ut Queant Laxis" and are believed to influence both the physical and spiritual aspects of an individual. While empirical scientific data might be scarce, proponents of Solfeggio frequencies suggest that these tones interact with the body's energy, promoting a harmonious state and influencing a person's emotional and physical well-being.

Exploring the Six Solfeggio Frequencies

- 174 Hz - Foundation and Security: This frequency creates a sense of security and safety. It's believed to facilitate fundamental changes and personal transformation, offering a stable base for inner growth.
- 285 Hz - Quantum Cognition and Expansion of Consciousness: This frequency is known for expanding consciousness and enabling greater mental clarity. It is also attributed to enhancing cognitive abilities and deepening self-awareness.
- 396 Hz - Liberating Guilt and Fear: Linked with the liberation from feelings of guilt and fear, this frequency assists in releasing negative emotions. It's associated with fostering a sense of security and inner peace.

- 417 Hz - "Undoing Situations and Facilitating Change" can be rephrased as "Reversing problematic situations and enabling progress."
- 528 Hz - Transformation and Miracles: Often called the "Love Frequency," 528 Hz is associated with transformation and miracles. It's believed to repair DNA and create harmony, bringing about profound changes and fostering love and compassion.
- 639 Hz - Connection and Relationships: This frequency is believed to enhance relationships and promote communication. It's associated with harmonizing interpersonal connections and resolving conflicts.

Each Solfeggio frequency is associated with unique attributes that address various aspects of human experience. The philosophical foundation suggests that by attuning oneself to these frequencies, individuals can access a path toward healing, spiritual elevation, and inner harmony.

While the tangible scientific evidence might be limited, the belief in the transformative power of these frequencies remains strong. Many practitioners and individuals exploring alternative healing methods find solace and support in these tones, using them as a pathway toward holistic well-being and spiritual growth.

Whether one embraces these frequencies as a spiritual tool or seeks comfort in their healing resonance, the Solfeggio frequencies continue to inspire a holistic approach to well-being, fostering a space for exploration, reflection, and potential transformation on a personal and spiritual level.

The 741 Hz frequency, often hailed as the "detoxifying frequency," holds the potential for aiding individuals battling chronic pain. In the realm of sound and vibrational therapy, this frequency is believed to possess unique healing properties, especially for those seeking relief from persistent pain.

This specific frequency, nestled within the Solfeggio scale, is attributed to the detoxification process. Advocates of sound therapy propose that exposure to 741 Hz could aid in releasing emotional or physical blockages, thereby contributing to a sense of relief and detoxification. While concrete scientific evidence supporting this frequency's direct impact on pain might be limited, many individuals exploring alternative healing methods find solace and potential relief through such vibrational therapies.

Chronic pain, a pervasive and often debilitating condition, impacts various aspects of an individual's life. The allure of vibrational therapy and frequencies like 741 Hz lies in their purported ability to ease these pains. Proponents suggest that this frequency aids in dissolving emotional blockages and promoting a sense of clarity, potentially resulting in a reduction of stress and, consequently, alleviating physical discomfort.

Using sound as a potential tool to address chronic pain is not a replacement for conventional medical treatment. However, for many individuals seeking complementary or alternative methods, exploring the potential benefits of sound therapy, including exposure to frequencies like 741 Hz, offers an additional dimension in their journey toward pain management.

Whether one sees sound frequencies as a spiritual aid or a complementary approach to conventional therapies, the notion of using sound as a potential avenue for relief from chronic pain continues to intrigue and inspire many. The vibrational nature of these frequencies invites an open-minded exploration into a holistic approach to well-being, providing a gentle and potentially impactful avenue for individuals striving to manage chronic pain and seeking a sense of relief and comfort.

As the understanding and appreciation of vibrational and sound therapy evolve, the potential of these frequencies, including 741 Hz, remains a fascinating area for ongoing exploration and investigation. This journey into sound's potential to alleviate chronic pain opens doors for personal and collective exploration, offering hope and potential relief to those seeking alternative avenues in their well-being.

The 852 Hz frequency is often associated with the amplification of intuition and spiritual guidance. Advocates of sound therapy suggest that exposure to 852 Hz could assist in awakening intuition, heightening self-awareness, and facilitating a deeper connection to the spiritual self. This frequency is believed to work on the spiritual level, encouraging awakening and inner strength.

On the other hand, 963 Hz is regarded as a frequency connected with the activation of the Pineal Gland, often referred to as the "God frequency" or the frequency of the gods. It is believed to enable individuals to achieve a state of unity and oneness, fostering a connection to the divine realm. Proponents of this frequency suggest that it allows for spiritual awakening and promotes a sense of enlightenment and pure connection to the universe.

While the tangible scientific evidence supporting the direct effects of these frequencies might be limited, many individuals exploring alternative healing methods find solace and potential personal growth through these frequencies. The essence of these frequencies lies in their potential to aid in pursuing spiritual growth and self-awareness.

Whether one embraces these frequencies as a spiritual tool or seeks enlightenment through their resonance, the potential effects of 852 Hz and 963 Hz continue to inspire and offer a pathway for personal exploration. As individuals continue to seek a deeper understanding of themselves and their connection to the spiritual realm, these frequencies stand as an avenue for potential growth and self-discovery.

Using Solfeggio frequencies effectively can offer a pathway to potential healing and relaxation. Here's a gentle guide to make the most of these frequencies:

- Selecting the Right Frequency: Choose the frequency that resonates most with your needs. Each frequency within the Solfeggio scale carries unique attributes. For instance, 396 Hz is associated with releasing fear and guilt, while 528 Hz is known as the "Love Frequency."
- Relax in a Calm Environment: Find a quiet and comfortable space where you won't be disturbed. Dim the lights, get cozy, and prepare to immerse yourself in the healing vibrations.

- Use Quality Headphones or Speakers: To fully experience the frequencies, use good quality headphones or speakers that accurately reproduce the tones. This allows for an immersive experience and better resonance.
- Set Intentions: Before listening, set your intentions. Whether it's stress relief, emotional healing, or relaxation, decide what you hope to achieve from the session.
- Repetitive Listening: Consistency is key. Regular and repeated exposure to these frequencies might yield more noticeable effects. Incorporate them into your routine during meditation, relaxation, or sleep.
- Openness and Patience: Embrace an open mind and a patient attitude. The effects might take time to notice, and results can vary. Allow yourself time to absorb and experience the frequencies.
- Mindfulness and Reflection: During and after listening, pay attention to how you feel. Reflect on any changes in your emotional or physical state. Journaling or noting your experiences can help track any shifts.
- Seek Professional Advice: While these frequencies are generally safe, listening in moderation is essential. Consult a healthcare professional before integrating these frequencies into your routine if you have any medical concerns or conditions.

Remember, these frequencies are not a substitute for professional medical treatment. They offer an additional avenue for relaxation and potential healing. Embrace these sounds as part of a holistic approach to well-being and allow them to complement your overall health routine.

CREATING YOUR HEALING PLAYLIST

The Therapeutic Power of Music for Fibromyalgia: Crafting Your Healing Playlist

In managing fibromyalgia, the journey toward healing often extends beyond conventional medicine. With its profound ability to touch the soul, music is a complementary tool in holistic healing. It offers solace, comfort, and a pathway toward emotional and mental well-being.

Holistic Healing: Integrating Music Therapy

While medicine addresses physical symptoms, music operates on a deeper level. It connects with emotions, serving as a balm for the soul. In the context of fibromyalgia, where emotional and mental well-being are crucial, music therapy emerges as a powerful complement to traditional treatments. It helps in managing stress, reducing anxiety, and elevating mood, fostering a holistic approach to healing.

Curating Your Therapeutic Playlist: A Step-by-Step Guide

Step 1: Reflect on Your Emotional State

Spend a moment reflecting on your feelings. Are you feeling anxious, sad, or perhaps hopeful? Identify your current emotional state.

Step 2: Select Tracks Reflecting Your Emotions

Choose 1 or 2 songs mirroring your current emotional state. These tracks should resonate with your feelings, offering a sense of validation and understanding. The key is to initiate your playlist with these tracks, creating a sense of alignment with your present emotional state. Then, transition gradually toward your desired emotional state with 3 or 4 subsequent tracks.

Step 3: Bridge from Current to Desired State

Select 3 or 4 songs that gradually shift in tone or tempo. These tracks act as a bridge, guiding you from your current emotional state toward your desired one.

Step 4: Choose Tracks Reflecting Your Desired Emotional State

Think about how you want to feel—energized, relaxed, or hopeful. Choose songs that evoke these emotions through their lyrics, melody, and rhythm. Explore different genres and artists; sometimes, a new genre might surprise you with its therapeutic effect.

Remember, personal resonance is key. If a song deeply connects with you and aids in your healing, it deserves a place on your playlist, regardless of others' opinions.

Crafting a therapeutic playlist involves a journey of self-discovery and emotional alignment. Let the melody guide you from your current emotional state toward a desired, more harmonious one. Through this process, music becomes a supportive and healing companion on your journey to manage fibromyalgia, offering solace, comfort, and a pathway toward emotional and mental well-being.

In *Sounds That Heal*, the power of music and sound therapy in managing fibromyalgia takes center stage. It explores the profound impact of music on emotional well-being and serves as a complement to conventional treatment. The chapter delves into creating personalized therapeutic playlists, tapping into the vibrant and healing potential of various frequencies and musical tones. It emphasizes the resonance between one's emotional state and music, guiding readers to curate playlists fostering emotional transitions and well-being.

Continuing on this journey of managing fibromyalgia, *Growth Amidst Pain* delves into the transformative power of mindset and personal development in navigating chronic conditions. This chapter ventures beyond the physical aspects, focusing on emotional resilience, coping strategies, and mental strength amid the challenges of chronic pain. It encourages a positive outlook and offers insights into fostering personal growth resilience and finding silver linings during the trials posed by chronic conditions. Join us as we explore the realm of emotional fortitude and personal evolution amidst the trials of chronic pain.

8

GROWTH AMIDST PAIN

> As for courage and will - we cannot measure how
> much of each lies within us; we can only trust
> there will be sufficient to carry through trials
> which may lie ahead.

— ANDRE NORTON

Growth amidst pain is a phrase that is often used to describe the process of overcoming adversity and becoming stronger as a result. It can be applied to many different areas of life, such as personal development, relationships, and careers. When you experience pain, seeing the situation's positive aspects cannot be easy. However, if you persevere through the pain, you can often emerge stronger and more resilient. Pain can teach you valuable lessons about yourself and the world around you. It can also help you to develop new skills and abilities.

In some cases, pain can lead to positive changes in your life. For example, it may motivate you to change your relationships, careers, or overall lifestyle. Ultimately, growth amidst pain reminds you that you can overcome anything life throws your way. If you are willing to face your pain head-on, you can learn from it stronger and more resilient than ever before.

Pain is a part of life, but it does not have to define who you are. You can choose to grow from your pain and become stronger as a result.

That sounds like an incredibly insightful chapter! Dealing with an invisible illness such as fibromyalgia can provide valuable insights and lessons for life. It is often a journey of self-discovery and resilience, allowing you to view your condition differently. Embracing the challenges and turning them into opportunities for personal growth and understanding can be incredibly empowering. The shift in perspective from seeing it solely as a challenge to recognizing it as a catalyst for growth is remarkable and can inspire many.

Living with fibromyalgia or any chronic condition can present numerous challenges that often test your endurance and resilience. If you have been on this journey, you have likely encountered moments of doubt, faced uphill battles, and found yourself delving deep into reservoirs of strength you might not have known existed.

In these trying times, it is important to acknowledge your incredible perseverance and courage. Reflect on the hurdles you have overcome, the small victories you have achieved, and the resilience you have shown despite the uncertainties. Each

step forward, no matter how small, is a testament to your unwavering strength.

Even when doubts lingered and the road seemed overwhelmingly tough, you've likely found unexpected wellsprings of determination and courage within yourself. There is immense power in acknowledging your strength, even when it feels faint.

Remember, you are not alone on this path. There is a community of people who understand and empathize with your journey. Sharing your experiences and seeking support can be a source of great solace and inspiration.

Embracing hope and empowerment is crucial. While the road may be challenging, it is also filled with opportunities for growth and self-discovery. Acknowledging the strength you have tapped into lays the foundation for a brighter, more empowered future.

So, take a moment to reflect on your journey, recognizing the strength and resilience that have carried you through. Celebrate your victories, no matter how small, and hold onto the hope that each step forward brings you closer to a place of greater strength and well-being. You are stronger than you think; your journey is a testament to your incredible fortitude. Remember that it is the little things that count.

REFRAMING FIBROMYALGIA

Chronic conditions like fibromyalgia can be challenging to manage and live with daily. However, by reframing how you perceive and approach these conditions through the lens of a growth mindset, you can empower yourself and transform your experience. A growth mindset involves embracing challenges and setbacks recognizing that abilities and talents can be developed through hard work and perseverance. Adopting this mindset can create new skills, coping mechanisms, and strategies to make a difference.

Growth Mindset vs. Fixed Mindset

A growth mindset involves believing dedication and hard work can develop abilities and qualities. It is about embracing new challenges, persisting in the face of setbacks, and seeing effort as the path to mastery. In contrast, a fixed mindset revolves around the belief that abilities are static and predetermined. People with a fixed mindset might intentionally steer clear of challenges and experience feelings of insecurity when confronted with the success of others.

Signs of a Fixed Mindset

Identifying a fixed mindset involves avoiding challenges, giving up easily, ignoring feedback, feeling threatened by others' success, and believing that effort is fruitless.

Importance of Developing the Right Mindset

Your mindset significantly influences your resilience, adaptability, and overall well-being. It affects how you face challenges, setbacks, and growth opportunities. For those with chronic conditions like fibromyalgia, developing a growth

mindset can be pivotal in managing the condition and leading a fulfilling life.

Impact of a Growth Mindset on Chronic Illness

A growth mindset in the context of chronic illness encourages seeing setbacks as opportunities for learning and adaptation. It involves understanding that the condition doesn't limit one's potential for growth. Embracing the belief that skills and abilities can be developed despite the illness's challenges is crucial.

Benefits of Nurturing Your Mindset

Nurturing a growth mindset can lead to increased resilience, reduced stress, improved coping mechanisms, and a more positive outlook. It can empower people to seek alternative strategies, focus on progress rather than perfection, and find meaning in their journey despite the challenges.

Strategies to Develop a Growth Mindset

- Owning Your Fear: Acknowledge the fears and uncertainties surrounding the condition, but do not let them define you. Recognize them as part of the journey and take steps to manage and overcome them.
- Embracing Discomfort: Accept that growth often occurs outside your comfort zone. Embrace discomfort as a sign of progress and an opportunity to adapt and grow.

- Accepting Setbacks as New Beginnings: View setbacks as learning experiences rather than failures. Embrace them as chances to discover new approaches and strategies for managing your condition.
- Realizing Life Is Not About Extremes: Recognize that progress isn't always linear. There will be ups and downs, but each experience contributes to your growth and learning.

We know that fibromyalgia can be a challenging condition to manage, but some people have managed to thrive despite the obstacles. These fibromyalgia warriors have applied a growth mindset to navigate the difficulties and have emerged stronger and more resilient. By sharing your real-life experiences, you can inspire others who are living with fibromyalgia to adopt a positive outlook and discover new ways to cope with the condition.

GRATITUDE IS THE ANCHOR IN LIFE'S STORMS

Gratitude can help you stay grounded and centered amid life's many challenges. It can remind you of the good things in your life and give you the strength to weather any storm. By expressing gratitude for what you have, you can cultivate inner peace and resilience to overcome tough times with positivity. So when the winds of change start blowing, remember that gratitude can be your anchor, providing stability and hope amidst the chaos.

Gratitude is an anchor in life's storms, especially for people managing fibromyalgia. This is not just feel-good advice; scientific evidence supports its profound benefits.

Research indicates that practicing gratitude significantly enhances the quality of life for individuals with fibromyalgia. By shifting the focus from what may be lacking to acknowledging and appreciating what's abundant, gratitude becomes a valuable positive psychological trait in this context.

To cultivate this powerful practice, here are three simple gratitude exercises that can be incorporated into daily life:

- Gratitude journaling: Spend a couple of minutes each day writing down things you are grateful for. These could be anything, from the sun's warmth on your face to the support of loved ones.
- Gratitude Letter: Write a letter expressing gratitude to someone who has positively impacted your life. This could be a friend, family member, or healthcare provider.
- Three Good Things Exercise: Each day, reflect on three good things that happened, regardless of their size. This practice helps shift focus towards the positive aspects of life.

By consistently engaging in these exercises, you can cultivate a habit of gratitude and improve your quality of life while navigating the challenges of fibromyalgia.

BEYOND THE FOG: FIBROMYALGIA'S HIDDEN LESSONS

Fibromyalgia's Hidden Lessons Beyond the Fog is a phrase that suggests that the chronic pain and fatigue experienced by those living with fibromyalgia have taught them valuable lessons that are not immediately apparent to others. The "fog" in this context refers to the brain fog that often accompanies fibromyalgia, making it difficult for sufferers to concentrate and think clearly. Despite the challenges they face, those who live with fibromyalgia often develop a resilience and strength that can inspire others.

Here are the empowering perspectives derived from living with fibromyalgia:

- You are stronger than you think: Despite the challenges, your resilience and endurance speak volumes about your inner strength and courage.
- Pain is not static: Recognize that pain fluctuates, reminding you that it's not permanent and that better moments are possible.
- Pain is a messenger: View pain as a signal, guiding you to pay attention to your body's needs and prompting necessary self-care and reflection.
- Pain is inevitable; suffering is optional: By understanding that while pain is a part of life, your reaction to it is within your control. You have the power to choose how it affects you.

- Asking for help opens the door for love: Seeking support isn't a sign of weakness but an act of courage that allows us to embrace the care and compassion of others.
- There is freedom in self-responsibility: Taking ownership of your well-being empowers you to make choices that prioritize your health and happiness.
- It's not your job to make others understand you: Your journey is yours; not everyone will comprehend it, and that's okay. Your focus should be on self-acceptance and growth.
- Falling apart can be liberating: Sometimes, allowing yourself to break down is the initial step towards healing and finding a renewed sense of freedom.

Remember, radical self-care is the birthplace of power. Nurturing yourself is not selfish but the cornerstone of your resilience and strength.

Lastly, know that your pain doesn't make you broken. You are whole. Your experiences, including pain, are a part of you, not something that diminishes your worth or completeness.

The main point of the chapter "Growth Amidst Pain" centers on the idea that personal growth often emerges from challenging or painful experiences. It explores how adversity can catalyze self-reflection, resilience, and personal development. The chapter highlights that while pain and difficulty can be distressing, they also offer learning, self-discovery, and growth opportunities.

GROWTH MINDSET IN FIBROMYALGIA

Coping with the emotional and physical pain and symptoms of fibromyalgia can take its toll and can be difficult, but there are ways to help maintain a positive outlook.

Engaging in gentle exercise can help reduce pain and improve well-being. Additionally, developing a support network of friends, family, and healthcare professionals can provide you with emotional support and help manage symptoms. Taking some time for self-care and the activities that bring you peace and relaxation is also important.

With the right support and self-care strategies, it is possible to live a fulfilling life with fibromyalgia.

However, there are ways to help maintain a positive outlook:

1. **Support System:** Surround yourself with understanding and supportive friends, family, or a support group. Having people who understand and empathize can make a significant difference.
2. **Mindfulness and Relaxation Techniques:** You can reduce your stress levels and improve your overall well-being by using mindfulness techniques such as meditation, deep breathing, yoga, and tai chi.
3. **Balanced Lifestyle:** Establish a routine that includes regular exercise, a balanced diet, and sufficient sleep. While it might be challenging, small and gentle movements or exercises suitable for your condition can make a difference.

4. **Pacing Activities:** Learn to pace yourself and manage your energy. Break tasks into smaller, manageable segments and take breaks as needed to avoid overexertion.

5. **Focus on What You Can Control:** Concentrate on things within your control. This can include your mindset, pain response, and self-care routine.

6. **Positive Distractions:** Engage in activities you enjoy or find fulfilling. This could be reading, hobbies, creative endeavors, or anything that brings you joy.

7. **Professional Support:** Work closely with healthcare providers, therapists, or counselors. They can provide strategies to cope with pain and help you navigate emotional challenges.

8. **Educate Yourself:** Understanding fibromyalgia better can help you feel more in control. Knowledge can also assist in explaining your condition to others.

9. **Practice Self-Compassion:** Be kind to yourself. Accept that there will be tough days, and don't be too hard on yourself when they happen.

Remember, everyone's journey is unique. It is important to find what works best for you in managing both the physical and emotional aspects of living with fibromyalgia. If you are struggling, seeking professional guidance is always a good idea.

EXERCISES

Life is full of challenges, and it's natural to feel overwhelmed and discouraged during tough times. However, choosing to embrace growth during these times can be a powerful journey. In the face of adversity, we focus on personal development and let go of fear. Building resilience and inner strength can help overcome obstacles. Through this growth process, you can learn valuable lessons and gain new perspectives that can positively impact your life in the long run.

Here are some exercises that can help you navigate and find growth amidst pain:

1. **Journaling:** Express your emotions, thoughts, and experiences. Reflect on the lessons you're learning during difficult times. Write about what you're grateful for or what gives you hope.

2. **Mindfulness and Meditation:** Practice mindfulness to stay present and acknowledge your feelings without judgment. Meditation can bring calmness and clarity, allowing you to focus on personal growth despite the pain.

3. **Seeking Support:** Talk to friends, family, or a professional. Sharing your experiences can provide different perspectives, comfort, and support and uncover solutions.

4. **Self-Compassion Exercises:** Treat yourself kindly. Practice self-compassion exercises to remind yourself that it's okay not to be perfect and to be kind to yourself during challenging times.

5. **Setting Goals:** Identify short-term and achievable goals that align with your growth. Even small steps forward can significantly impact personal development.

6. **Learning from Pain:** Explore the lessons and insights pain brings. Ask yourself what this experience teaches you and how it can contribute to your growth.
7. **Creativity and Expression:** Engage in creative activities that help you express your emotions. Creativity, whether expressed through painting, writing, or music, can be therapeutic and aid growth.
8. **Physical Exercise:** Take care of your body. Physical activity boosts your mood and helps manage stress, allowing you to focus on personal development.

Remember, growth in the face of pain is a unique and personal journey. Be patient and kind to yourself throughout the process. If you're going through a challenging time, seeking help from a professional can be immensely helpful.

Coping with the progression of fibromyalgia while maintaining a positive outlook can indeed be daunting. The constant battle against pain and the uncertainties that come with its progression can feel overwhelming. However, it's crucial to understand that while fibromyalgia is a part of your life, it doesn't define who you are. Here are some ways to stay positive despite the challenges it presents.

Firstly, cultivating a positive mindset is vital. We can find a path towards a fulfilling life by acknowledging pain and focusing on joy and contentment. Find activities or hobbies that bring you happiness and peace, whether reading, painting, listening to music, or spending time with loved ones. These moments of joy can act as powerful counterweights to difficult times.

Additionally, educating yourself about fibromyalgia can be empowering. Understanding your condition, its triggers, and how to manage it can provide a sense of control. Knowledge often leads to better management and a more positive outlook.

Support networks are invaluable. Connecting with others who understand what you're going through can offer immense comfort. Whether it's a support group, online community, or close friends and family, sharing experiences and strategies for coping can alleviate feelings of isolation and provide a source of strength.

Practice self-care regularly. It is important to prioritize your mental, physical, and emotional health. This means taking steps to ensure that you are taking care of yourself in all aspects, including exercise, healthy eating, and seeking professional help if needed. Simple practices like gentle exercises, mindfulness, adequate sleep, and a healthy diet can make a substantial difference in managing your symptoms and boosting your overall mood.

Setting realistic goals is another positive step forward. Break down tasks into more manageable tasks and celebrate each small achievement. This not only gives you a sense of accomplishment but also serves as a reminder of your resilience and determination in the face of adversity.

Keep an open line of communication with your healthcare provider. A strong partnership with your doctor ensures you receive the best possible treatment. Exploring different therapies or medications may help manage symptoms, which can enhance your quality of life.

It's crucial to accept both good and bad days. Acknowledge your feelings and allow yourself to experience them fully without judgment. It's okay not to be okay sometimes. Embracing this reality can release some of the mental pressure and offer a more balanced perspective.

Remember, your health condition does not determine your worth. You are a valuable person who can contribute positively to the world around you. Cherish the things that make you unique and focus on your strengths.

While living with fibromyalgia can present its share of challenges, it's essential to recognize that there is still much beauty and joy to be found in life. Your strength, resilience, and capacity for positivity despite the pain are truly commendable. You're not alone in this journey; with the right strategies and support, it's possible to find moments of happiness and contentment along the way.

It is a logical continuation of the chapter's discussion about growth. Here, it may reflect on how the people or stories discussed in the chapter have transformed, adapted, and emerged stronger after navigating through their painful experiences. The conclusion could emphasize the importance of recognizing the potential for growth in times of struggle and how embracing these challenges can lead to personal development and newfound strength. It also encourages readers to view difficulties as opportunities for growth rather than solely as setbacks.

CONCLUSION

Fibromyalgia Unraveled is a book that offers valuable insights into the disease, its symptoms, and the various treatment options available. To truly understand the book's essence, one must focus on its core messages rather than every single detail. You can apply the knowledge gained to improve their lives by understanding this invisible illness more deeply. The revelations found within the book's pages provide a powerful foundation for moving forward, helping readers manage their symptoms better and improve their quality of life.

As you conclude your journey through *Fibromyalgia Unraveled*, remember that knowledge is power. This book aimed to untangle the complexities of fibromyalgia, offering insights, strategies, and support. While it's a condition that brings challenges, it's essential to remember that you are not defined by it. Your resilience, the ability to find joy in small victories, and the strength to navigate each day are the true markers of your story. Embrace each moment, seek support when needed, and remember that life, despite its hurdles, remains a beautiful journey worth celebrating. Your journey with fibromyalgia is unique, but you're never alone in it.

KEY TAKEAWAYS

Listening to Your Body's Language: The book emphasized the importance of tuning into your body's signals. Understanding these messages can profoundly impact your management of fibromyalgia, empowering you to respond effectively to its cues.

The Impact of Lifestyle Choices: From the significance of rest to the healing potential of movement, the book highlighted how lifestyle adjustments, especially in nutrition and activity, can significantly influence your journey with fibromyalgia.

Creating Your Sanctuary: It highlighted the importance of establishing a supportive environment. Your physical or emotional sanctuary acts as a haven where healing, comfort, and peace prevail.

Growth Amidst Pain: One of the most empowering messages revolved around finding strength and wisdom amidst the challenges of chronic pain. It reframed the experience of fibromyalgia as an opportunity for personal growth and resilience.

CLOSING AFFIRMATIONS:

Now, take a moment to embrace the affirmations that uplift, inspire, and empower you:

- Your strength surpasses any limitation.
- Your journey with fibromyalgia is unique, and you're in control.
- Every small victory counts; celebrate each moment.
- Your pain doesn't define you; you are whole beyond it.
- Embrace self-care as an act of personal empowerment.
- Seek support and love in asking for help.
- There's wisdom and growth in every challenge you face.
- You are not alone; your journey matters.

And always remember:

- Fibromyalgia can be challenging to manage, but it is important to remember that it doesn't define who you are as a person. You are more than your fibromyalgia. You have unique talents, skills, and qualities that make you who you are, and fibromyalgia is just one aspect of your life. While it may require some adjustments and accommodations to manage your symptoms, focusing on the things that bring you joy and fulfillment is crucial. Remember, fibromyalgia may be a part of you, but it isn't all of you.
- Life is full of ups and downs, challenges and triumphs, but it remains a precious and beautiful gift. Whether you're experiencing a moment of relief from a difficult

situation or basking in the glow of a major achievement, it's important to take a moment to celebrate and appreciate the good things in life. So, take the time to cherish and savor every moment, big or small, and remember that life is truly something to be grateful for.

Living with fibromyalgia can be a challenging and often unpredictable journey. That's why it's important to have affirmations and reminders to keep you motivated and focused on your path. These affirmations can remind you that you are strong and resilient and that you have the ability to face any obstacle that comes your way. It's also important to remember that even in the midst of your struggles, there are moments of joy and celebration that are worth cherishing.

Often, it's the simple things that bring us the greatest joy in life. Spending time with the people we care about, pursuing our favorite hobbies, and achieving small goals can all be incredibly fulfilling experiences. These moments may seem insignificant, but they have the power to brighten our days and bring us a sense of happiness and contentment that can last long after the moment has passed. Therefore, it's important to cherish these moments and make time for them in our busy lives. While it's easy to feel isolated and alone in your journey, it's important to remember that you are not alone. Many others are on a similar journey, and resources and support are available to help you along the way. So, as you navigate your unique journey with fibromyalgia, keep these affirmations and reminders close to your heart.

Embrace your strength and resilience, seek out moments of joy and celebration, and remember that you are not alone. Your journey is worth celebrating, and you have the power to create a fulfilling and meaningful life despite the challenges that may arise.

Your Voice, Their Beacon

As you turn the final pages of "Fibromyalgia Unraveled," you're now armed with knowledge, strategies, and a renewed sense of hope in your battle against fibromyalgia. But your journey doesn't end here – in fact, a new chapter begins, one where you can be a guiding light for others.

Your insights and experiences are invaluable. By sharing your honest thoughts about this book on Amazon, you do so much more than just write a review. You become a part of someone else's journey, guiding them to the help and understanding they desperately seek.

Every review is a beacon of hope for other Fibro Warriors. It's a way to pass on the torch of knowledge and support, showing others where they can find the same resources and encouragement that have helped you. Your words have the power to uplift, to inspire, and to empower.

We're all in this fight together, and every bit of knowledge shared keeps the hope alive for those still searching for answers. Your contribution, your voice, matters immensely.

Ready to make an impact? Scan the QR code below to leave your review on Amazon and light the way for someone else on their path to healing and understanding.

Nadal-Nicolás, Y., Miralles-Amorós, L., Martínez-Olcina, M., Sánchez-Ortega, M., Mora, J., & Martínez-Rodríguez, A. (2021). Vegetarian and vegan diet in fibromyalgia: A systematic review. *International Journal of Environmental Research and Public Health, 18*(9), 4955. https://doi.org/10.3390/ijerph18094955

O'Sullivan, S. (2017, January 3). *When the body speaks.* Psychology Today. https://www.psychologytoday.com/us/articles/201701/when-the-body-speaks

Our body talks to us through pain and sickness. (2018, January 4). Exploring Your Mind. https://exploringyourmind.com/body-talks-through-pain-sickness

Pattemore, C. (2022, August 5). *Spending time in nature is good for you. new research explains why.* Healthline. https://www.healthline.com/health-news/spending-time-in-nature-is-good-for-you-new-research-explains-why

Penn, I.-W., Chuang, E., Chuang, T.-Y., Lin, C.-L., & Kao, C.-H. (2019). Bidirectional association between migraine and fibromyalgia: Retrospective cohort analyses of two populations. *BMJ Open, 9*(4), e026581. https://doi.org/10.1136/bmjopen-2018-026581

Peres), M. P. (Mikey. (2022, January 26). *Your energy is like currency. invest it wisely to see the greatest rewards.* Entrepreneur. https://www.entrepreneur.com/growing-a-business/your-energy-is-like-currency-invest-it-wisely-to-see-the/411677

Perry, E. (2021, December 1). *Is your brain tired? Here are six ways to treat mental fatigue.* Better Up. https://www.betterup.com/blog/mental-fatigue

Phillips, Q. (2022, July 26). *Ten myths and facts about fibromyalgia | everyday health.* EverydayHealth.com. https://www.everydayhealth.com/fibromyalgia/myths-facts-about-fibromyalgia/

Priya, A. (2022, October 29). *The concept of healing spaces.* RTF | Rethinking the Future. https://www.re-thinkingthefuture.com/designing-for-typologies/a8342-the-concept-of-healing-spaces/

Rabois, I. (2018, August 12). *Mindful listening in a noisy world.* Mindful Teachers. https://www.mindfulteachers.org/blog/mindful-listening-in-a-noisy-world

Regan, S. (2022, February 27). *A quick practice for relieving stress & tension — anytime, anywhere.* Mindbodygreen. https://www.mindbodygreen.com/articles/body-scan-meditation-how-it-works-benefits-tips-more

Ruijter, I. de. (2020, March 3). *Body signals: Are you listening?* Mindfulness-

Project. https://www.mindfulness-project.org/2020/03/03/body-signals-are-you-listening/

Sebastien, T. R. (2018, January 18). *Longing for quiet in a noisy world: How I found myself & peace in silence*. Tiny Buddha. https://tinybuddha.com/blog/longing-for-quiet-in-a-noisy-world-how-i-found-myself-and-peace-in-silence/

Sleep, B. (2019a, May 31). *How binaural beats affect your brain | bettersleep*. Better Sleep. https://www.bettersleep.com/blog/how-binaural-beats-affect-your-brain/

Sleep, B. (2019b, December 16). *The science behind solfeggio frequencies | bettersleep*. Www.bettersleep.com. https://www.bettersleep.com/blog/science-behind-solfeggio-frequencies/

Smith, L. (2022, September 1). *Seven people with fibromyalgia describe what it feels like*. GoodRx. https://www.goodrx.com/conditions/fibromyalgia/what-fibromyalgia-feels-like

Sound healing 101: The science behind sound healing. (n.d.). Masterpeacebox. Retrieved November 10, 2023, from https://www.masterpeacebox.com/post/sound-healing-101-the-science-behind-sound-healing-how-to-practice-at-home

Stephens, S. (2018, March 16). *Exercise and fibromyalgia: Yes, you should*. EverydayHealth.com. https://www.everydayhealth.com/fibromyalgia/treatment/exercise-fibromyalgia-yes-you-should/

Stephens, S. (2022, September 26). *Fibromyalgia: What to eat, what to avoid*. EverydayHealth.com. https://www.everydayhealth.com/fibromyalgia/diet/fibromyalgia-what-eat-what-avoid/

Story, C. M. (2021, March 9). *How a mindfulness practice can help ease fibromyalgia pain*. Healthline. https://www.healthline.com/health/fibromyalgia-mindfulness

Sulivan, D. (2023, July 25). *Symptoms journaling: What, why, and how*. Healthline. https://www.healthline.com/health/symptoms-journal

Suni, E. (2020, October 23). *How sleep works: Understanding the science of sleep*. Sleep Foundation. https://www.sleepfoundation.org/how-sleep-works

The benefits of gratitude when living with a chronic illness. (2021, January 25). Bezzy MS. https://www.bezzyms.com/discover/mental-well-being-ms/health-the-benefits-of-gratitude-when-you're-living-with-a-chronic-illness

The complete guide to sound baths and sound bathing therapy. (2019). Shanti Bowl.

https://www.shantibowl.com/blogs/blog/guide-to-sound-baths-and-sound-bathing-therapy

Tinsley, G. (2021, February 28). *What to eat or avoid to ease your fibromyalgia symptoms.* Healthline. https://www.healthline.com/health/fibromyalgia-diet-to-ease-symptoms#the-bottom-line

ucmsocialmediateam. (2019, August 11). *Five tips and tricks to manage fibromyalgia fatigue.* Tranquility Specific Chiropractic. https://tschiropractic.com/2019/08/11/5-tips-and-tricks-to-manage-fibromyalgia-fatigue

Victor, D. (2023, April 3). *Music as A universal language of healing - harmony & healing.* Harmouny & Healing. https://www.harmonyandhealing.org/music-as-a-universal-language-of-healing/

Weir, K. (2020, April 1). Nurtured by nature. *American Psychological Association, 51*(3). https://www.apa.org/monitor/2020/04/nurtured-nature

What is earthing grounding & can it transform your health? (2015). Betterearthing.com.au. https://betterearthing.com.au/what-is-earthing/

Wickerson, N. (n.d.). *A boost by better breathing.* UK Fibromyalgia Magazine. Retrieved November 10, 2023, from https://ukfibromyalgia.com/blog/a-boost-by-better-breathingCelebrating

Thank you for being a vital part of this community. Your involvement doesn't just help keep the fight against fibromyalgia alive; it helps it thrive.

Together, we are stronger. Let's continue to share, support, and inspire.

Courtney Dale, alongside the entire Fibro Warrior community

REFERENCES

A quote from Celebrating Silence: Life-changing. (n.d.). Www.goodreads.com. Retrieved November 10, 2023, from https://www.goodreads.com/quotes/ 401577-activity-and-rest-are-two-vital-aspects-of-life-to

Andersson, U. M., Åberg, A. C., von Koch, L., & Palstam, A. (2021). Women with fibromyalgia prefer resistance exercise with heavy loads—a randomized crossover pilot study. *International Journal of Environmental Research and Public Health, 18*(12), 6276. https://doi.org/10.3390/ijerph18126276

Anna. (2015, July 5). *The life-changing silence*: Life-changing *lessons I (reluctantly) learned from chronic pain.* Anna Lovind. https://annalovind.com/ok-pain-what-have-you-got-for-me-the-life-changing-lessons-i-reluctantly-learned-from-chronic-pain/

April 8, H. E. U., Development, 2021 C. P., Productivity, & Relaxation. (2007, September 18). *9 things you can do tonight to prepare for tomorrow.* The Positivity Blog. https://www.positivityblog.com/9-things-you-can-do-tonight-to-prepare-for-tomorrow/

Boskey, E. (2023, March 24). *What is a negative feedback loop?* Verywell Health; Verywellhealth. https://www.verywellhealth.com/what-is-a-negative-feedback-loop-3132878

Boughton, T. (2019, September 3). *Fibromyalgia triggers.* News-Medical.net. https://www.news-medical.net/health/Fibromyalgia-Triggers.aspx

Bruce, D. F., & Ph.DFibrofog. (2022, August 4). *The benefits of exercise for fibromyalgia.* WebMD. https://www.webmd.com/fibromyalgia/fibromyalgia-and-exercise

Canter, J. (2021, August 11). *Fibrofog and fatigue.* WebMD. https://www.webmd.com/fibromyalgia/fibromyalgia-and-fatigue

Chen, K., Zhang, T., Liu, F., Zhang, Y., & Song, Y. (2021). How Does Urban Green Space Impact Residents' Mental Health: A Literature Review of Mediators. *International Journal of Environmental Research and Public Health, 18*(22), 11746. https://doi.org/10.3390/ijerph182211746

Cherney, K. (2014). *Fibromyalgia: Causes, trigger points, treatment, and more.* Healthline. https://www.healthline.com/health/fibromyalgia

Cherry, K. (2019, December 10). *How listening to music can have psychological benefits.* Verywell Mind. https://www.verywellmind.com/surprising-psychological-benefits-of-music-4126866

Clements, J. (2022, July 8). *Seven exercises to ease fibromyalgia pain.* GoodRx; GoodRx. https://www.goodrx.com/conditions/fibromyalgia/exercises-to-help-manage-fibromyalgia-pain

Dellwo, A. (2022, May 25). *How to pace yourself without overdoing it when you have fibromyalgia.* Verywell Health. https://www.verywellhealth.com/pacing-yourself-with-fibromyalgia-and-mecfs-715723

Dellwo, A. (2013, September 11). *The seven types of fibromyalgia pain.* Verywell Health. https://www.verywellhealth.com/seven-types-of-fibromyalgia-pain-716138

Dellwo, A. (2014, December 23). *The challenges of weight loss with fibromyalgia.* Verywell Health; Verywell Health. https://www.verywellhealth.com/weight-loss-fibromyalgia-the-challenges-715789

Dellwo, A. (2019). *A day in my life with fibromyalgia.* Verywell Health. https://www.verywellhealth.com/a-day-in-my-life-with-fibromyalgia-715591

Dellwo, A. (2022a, June 5). *Is fibromyalgia caused by gut bacteria?* Verywell Health. https://www.verywellhealth.com/fibromyalgia-gut-microbiome-4774803

Dellwo, A. (2022b, June 30). *What to eat if you have fibromyalgia.* Verywell Health. https://www.verywellhealth.com/fibromyalgia-diet-good-and-bad-foods-4144693

Dr LaPuma. (2019, July 16). *Listening when your body talks | healthy living, wellness & nutrition expert | Dr. John la Puma.* Dr. John La Puma. https://www.drjohnlapuma.com/wellness-and-health/listening-when-your-body-talks/

Exercise and fibromyalgia healthlink BC. (2023, September 25). Www.healthlinkbc.ca. https://www.healthlinkbc.ca/healthy-eating-physical-activity/conditions/exercise-and-fibromyalgia

Field, B. (2021, July 21). *What is forest bathing?* Verywell Mind. https://www.verywellmind.com/what-is-forest-bathing-5190723

Fishman, R. (2020, November 22). *Your body is speaking to you - renée fishman.* My Meadow Report. https://mymeadowreport.com/reneefishman/2020/your-body-is-speaking-to-you

Franz Martín, Blanco-Suárez, M., Zambrano, P., Cáceres, O., Almirall, M., Alegre, J., Lobo, B., González-Castro, A. M., Santos, J., Joan Carles Domingo, Jurek, J., & Jesús Castro-Marrero. (2023). Increased gut permeability and bacterial translocation are associated with fibromyalgia and myalgic encephalomyelitis/chronic fatigue syndrome: Implications for disease-related biomarker discovery. *Frontiers in Immunology, 14.* https://doi.org/10.3389/fimmu.2023.1253121

Gould, W. R. (2023, March 3). *What are sound baths?* Verywell Mind. https://www.verywellmind.com/what-are-sound-baths-4783501

Haagenson, K. (2020, December 15). *How A growth mindset makes you more powerful - femmepower blog.* Femme Power. https://www.femmepowerblog.com/personal-growth/growth-mindset

Hoffer, M. (2022, December 2). *How music affects your mind, mood and body.* Www.tmh.org. https://www.tmh.org/healthy-living/blogs/healthy-living/how-music-affects-your-mind-mood-and-body#:~:

How does fibromyalgia affect emotional health?: Pain medicine consultants: Pain specialists. (n.d.). Www.painmedicineconsultants.com. Retrieved November 1, 2023, from https://www.painmedicineconsultants.com/blog/how-does-fibromyalgia-affect-emotional-health

How to use solfeggio frequencies – powerthoughts meditation club. (n.d.). Power Thoughts. Retrieved November 10, 2023, from https://power thoughtsmeditationclub.com/how-to-use-solfeggio-frequencies/

Ibe, O. (2023, May 4). *What is earthing?* Verywell Mind. https://www.verywell mind.com/what-is-earthing-5220089

Knight, M. (2020, September 26). *Technique: Keeping an energy diary.* Leapers. https://medium.com/leapers/technique-keeping-an-energy-diary-4d59fe9a39f8

Koller, T. (2017, June 1). *Mindset changes I made as a chronic illness reshaped my life.* Thrive Global. https://medium.com/thrive-global/mindset-changes-i-made-as-a-chronic-illness-reshaped-my-life-ffbfb44b2a56

Kumar, K. (n.d.). *What foods trigger fibromyalgia pain? Diet & nutrition.* MedicineNet. Retrieved November 10, 2023, from https://www.medicinenet.com/what_foods_trigger_fibromyalgia_pain/article.htm

Lawrenz, L. (2023, August 17). *Binaural beats: Benefits and tips for use.* Psych Central. https://psychcentral.com/health/binaural-beats

Lindberg, S. (2023, March 23). *How your environment affects your mental health.* Verywell Mind. https://www.verywellmind.com/how-your-environment-affects-your-mental-health-5093687

Living with fibromyalgia: Pet assisted therapy. (2014, August 2). The Fibroclinic. https://www.thefibroclinic.com/pet-assisted-therapy/

Lumen Learning. (2019). *Homeostasis and feedback loops | anatomy and physiology I*. Lumenlearning.com. https://courses.lumenlearning.com/suny-ap1/chapter/homeostasis-and-feedback-loops/

Mandal, A. (2013, June 3). *Fibromyalgia epidemiology*. News-Medical.net. https://www.news-medical.net/health/Fibromyalgia-Epidemiology.aspx

Marina. (2022, March 25). *Top 7 best chronic illness symptom tracker apps in 2022*. The Discerning You. https://thediscerningyou.com/chronic-illness-symptom-tracker-apps/

May, B. (2021, March 19). *Fibromyalgia linked to hypersensitivity to heat and auditory stimuli*. Clinical Pain Advisor. https://www.clinicalpainadvisor.com/musculoskeletal-pain/fibromyalgia-may-cause-hypersensitivity-to-heat-and-sound-as-well-as-pain/

Mayo Clinic. (2017). *Fibromyalgia - diagnosis and treatment - Mayo Clinic*. Mayo Clinic. https://www.mayoclinic.org/diseases-conditions/fibromyalgia/diagnosis-treatment/drc-20354785

Mayo Clinic. (2021, October 26). *Fibromyalgia*. Mayo Clinic. https://www.mayoclinic.org/diseases-conditions/fibromyalgia/symptoms-causes/syc-20354780

Mayo Clinic Staff. (2018). *10 great reasons to love aerobic exercise*. Mayo Clinic. https://www.mayoclinic.org/healthy-lifestyle/fitness/in-depth/aerobic-exercise/art-20045541

MCLOUGHLIN, M. J., COLBERT, L. H., STEGNER, A. J., & COOK, D. B. (2011). Are women with fibromyalgia less physically active than healthy women? *Medicine & Science in Sports & Exercise, 43*(5), 905–912. https://doi.org/10.1249/mss.0b013e3181fca1ea

Mehta, S. (2023, May). *The body gives warning signals; don't ignore them*. Deccan Chronicle; Deccan Chronicle. https://www.deccanchronicle.com/lifestyle/health-and-wellbeing/010523/the-body-gives-warning-signals-dont-ignore-them.html

Menchaca, D. (2020, February 20). *5 apps for symptom diary & health journaling (2020)*. Www.teamscopeapp.com. https://www.teamscopeapp.com/blog/5-diary-apps-for-tracking-symptoms

Mind. (2021, November). *How nature benefits mental health*. Www.mind.org.uk. https://www.mind.org.uk/information-support/tips-for-everyday-living/nature-and-mental-health/how-nature-benefits-mental-health/

MindTools | home. (n.d.). Www.mindtools.com. Retrieved November 10, 2023, from https://www.mindtools.com/adwtc03/prioritization